P9-DUM-800

ACCOUNTING FUNDAMENTALS
FOR
HEALTH CARE MANAGEMENT

WITHDRAWN
UTSA LIBRARIES

Steven A. Finkler, PhD, CPA
Professor of Public and Health Administration,
Accounting, and Financial Management
The Robert F. Wagner Graduate School of Public Service
New York University
New York, NY

David M. Ward, PhD
Professor of Health Administration and Policy
College of Health Professions
Medical University of South Carolina
Charleston, SC

JONES AND BARTLETT PUBLISHERS
Sudbury, Massachusetts
BOSTON   TORONTO   LONDON   SINGAPORE

World Headquarters

Jones and Bartlett Publishers
40 Tall Pine Drive
Sudbury, MA 01776
978-443-5000
info@jbpub.com
www.jbpub.com

Jones and Bartlett Publishers
Canada
6339 Ormindale Way
Mississauga, Ontario L5V 1J2
CANADA

Jones and Bartlett Publishers
International
Barb House, Barb Mews
London W6 7PA
UK

Jones and Bartlett's books and products are available through most bookstores and online booksellers. To contact Jones and Bartlett Publishers directly, call 800-832-0034, fax 978-443-8000, or visit our website www.jbpub.com.

Substantial discounts on bulk quantities of Jones and Bartlett's publications are available to corporations, professional associations, and other qualified organizations. For details and specific discount information, contact the special sales department at Jones and Bartlett via the above contact information or send an email to specialsales@jbpub.com.

Copyright © 2006 by Jones and Bartlett Publishers, Inc.

ISBN-13: 978-0-7637-2675-1

ISBN-10: 0-7637-2675-3

All rights reserved. No part of the material protected by this copyright may be reproduced or utilized in any form, electronic or mechanical, including photocopying, recording, or by any information storage and retrieval system, without written permission from the copyright owner.

Library of Congress Cataloging-in-Publication Data
Finkler, Steven A.
   Accounting fundamentals for health care management / Steven A.
Finkler, David M. Ward.
      p. cm.
   Includes bibliographical references and index.
   ISBN-13: 978-0-7637-2675-1 (pbk.)
   1. Integrated delivery of health care. 2. Health services adminis-
tration. 3. Public health administration.   I. Ward, David M.
II. Title.
   [DNLM: 1. Delivery of Health Care, Integrated—economics.
2. Health Services Administration—economics. 3. Public Health
Administration—economics. 4. Financial Management—methods.
W 84.1 F503a 2006]
RA971.F52 2006
362.1068—dc22

                                        2005029504

6048

Production Credits
Publisher: Michael Brown
Associate Editor: Kylah Goodfellow McNeill
Production Director: Amy Rose
Associate Production Editor: Daniel Stone
Associate Marketing Manager: Marissa Hederson
Manufacturing Buyer: Therese Connell
Composition: Arlene Apone
Cover Design: Kristin E. Ohlin
Printing and Binding: Malloy, Inc.
Cover Printing: Malloy, Inc.

Printed in the United States of America
10 09 08 07 06   10 9 8 7 6 5 4 3 2 1

Library
University of Texas
at San Antonio

Dedication

In Memory of Joe and Shirley Finkler
and
To Howard and Marilyn Ward

Acknowledgments

Portions of this text have been reprinted/adapted with permission from *Finance and Accounting for Nonfinancial Managers, Third Edition,* Steven A. Finkler, Aspen Publishers, Copyright 2003, pages 3-7, 9-10, 29-34, 35-38, 40-42, 43-58, 59-69, 71-76, 78-93, 95-97, 99-102, 104-105, 125-134, 167-182, 189-202, 203-235, 263-264, 266-269, 271-272, 274-277, 287, 290, and 292-309.

Contents

Preface

The complexity of today's health care system has brought with it a need for all managers and executives to have a solid understanding of accounting. This book is geared toward the student or current health care manager who needs a basic grounding in financial accounting within health care organizations. It is presented from the basic premise that knowledge of accounting is beneficial regardless of a person's primary focus within the health care system. The operating room nurse, the compliance officer, the physician practice manager, or the pharmaceutical sales representative, can all benefit from a better understanding of health care accounting.

This book will not make anyone a chief financial officer. It will, however, provide the vocabulary and introduction to the tools and concepts employed by finance officers. It will help the nonfinancial manager assess financial information, ask the appropriate questions, and understand the jargon-laden answers.

To help enable the use of this book within the framework of a health care accounting course, we have posted end-of-chapter questions and problems on the book's Web site at www.jbpub.com/catalog/0763726753. In addition, the Web site includes a number of Excel templates that can help the reader use the various tools presented in the book.

We have attempted to cover the material in a thorough yet not overwhelming manner. However, we recognize that there is always room for improvement. Readers are encouraged to use the Web page (www.jbpub.com/catalog/0763726753) to e-mail us to point out errors or unclear passages, or to suggest additional applications or other improvements. All contributions will be acknowledged in the next edition. Any corrections to errors in the text will be posted on the Web page.

The authors wish to thank Daniel Stone, Michael Brown, and Kylah McNeil from Jones and Bartlett Publishers for all their help in bringing this book from conception to reality.

Steven A. Finkler
David M. Ward

The companion Web site for this book contains Excel templates available for download. These templates have been designed to help the reader use various tools illustrated in the text of this book. PowerPoint slides and end-of-chapter questions have also been posted to this site. To access the supplemental material for this text on the Web, please visit:

http://www.jbpub.com/catalog/0763726753/supplements.htm.

CHAPTER 1

Introduction to Health Care Accounting and Financial Management

DO I REALLY NEED TO UNDERSTAND ACCOUNTING TO BE EFFECTIVE IN MY HEALTH CARE ORGANIZATION?

Today's health care system, with its many different types of health care organizations, is extremely complex. The science of health care is complex, the physical maintenance of the facilities is complex, the interactions and human behaviors within the organizations are complex, and so too are the financial and accounting requirements. The complexity of today's environment has resulted in the spread of accounting and financial management to all areas within a health care organization. Accounting and financial management is no longer the sole purview of the finance department. Nurse-managers are being held responsible for the financial management of their units, pharmacy directors are making significant financial management decisions on a daily basis, operating room (OR) managers must maintain efficient utilization rates and keep patients flowing through the OR to maintain the financial health of the organization.

To be successful, health care managers and executives (regardless of what specific area within a health care organization they lead) must all have a firm understanding of ac-counting and financial management. It is clear that not everyone will become the Chief Financial Officer, but everyone is making financial decisions and needs to be able to communicate effectively with financial managers.

WHAT IS FINANCIAL MANAGEMENT?

This book focuses on health care accounting and finance (Figure 1-1). *Accounting* is a system for providing financial information. It is generally broken down into two principal elements: financial accounting and managerial accounting. *Finance* has traditionally been thought of as the area of financial management that supervises the acquisition and disposition of the organization's resources, especially cash.

The *financial accounting* aspect of accounting is a formalized system designed to record

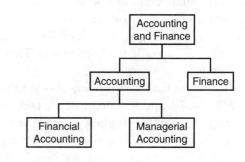

Figure 1-1 Accounting and Finance

the financial history of the health care organization. The financial accountant is simply a historian who uses dollar signs. An integral part of the financial accountant's job is to report the organization's history from time to time to interested individuals, usually through the organization's quarterly and annual reports.

The *managerial accountant* looks forward; the financial accountant looks backward. Instead of reporting on what has happened, the managerial accountant provides financial information that might be used for making improved decisions regarding the future. In many organizations the same individual is responsible for providing both financial and managerial accounting information.

Finance has expanded significantly from the functions of borrowing funds and investing the excess cash resources of the firm. In its broader sense, the finance function involves providing financial analyses to improve decisions that affect the wealth of the organization. Whereas the managerial accountant provides the information for use in the analyses, the finance officer often performs the actual analyses.

WHAT ARE THE GOALS OF FINANCIAL MANAGEMENT WITHIN HEALTH CARE ORGANIZATIONS?

At first, one might simply say that the goal of financial management is to aid in the maximization of wealth, or more simply, maximization of the organization's profits. Profits are, after all, literally, the bottom line. That is true, but as managers know, the health care environment has many other goals—improving the health and well-being of the community, providing the highest quality health care services, and minimizing morbidity and mortality, for example. For many health care organizations (e.g., not-for-profit hospitals)

maximization of profit may not be a goal at all, although at least some profit is usually necessary to ensure the financial well-being of even these organizations.

On a more personal level, managers are concerned with maximization of salaries and benefits. In a for-profit organization, such maximization is often tied in with the maximization of return on investments (ROI), return on equity (ROE), return on assets (ROA), or return on net assets (RONA) (see Chapter 13). The list of goals within the organization is relatively endless, and our intention is to narrow the range rather than broaden it.

From the perspective of financial management there are two overriding goals: profitability and viability (Figure 1-2). The organization wants to be profitable and it wants to continue in business. It is possible to be profitable and yet fail to continue in business. Both goals require some clarification and additional discussion because they surface from time to time throughout this book.

Profitability

As stated, many health care organizations do not have the maximization of profit as a goal but they must generate some level of profit in order to achieve their other goals. Whether for profit or not for profit, health care organizations need profits to invest in expansion of services so there is wider access to health care. Health care organizations need profits so they can acquire new technologies to improve the

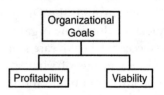

Figure 1-2 Organizational Goals

quality of health care. And health care organizations need profits to replace old buildings and equipment as they wear out. Generally, replacement facilities are more expensive than the ones they replace, because of inflation if nothing else, and profits are used to cover some of those higher costs. Because of this, we continue to use the terms *profit* and *profitability,* even when referring to not-for-profit health care organizations.

This does not mean that profits are the only goal. They are not even always the primary goal. High-quality health care often comes first. However, we must always bear in mind that profits are necessary to be able to achieve the goals related to providing high-quality care.

In maximizing profits, there is always a trade-off with risk (Figure 1-3). The greater the risk we must incur, the greater the anticipated profit or return on our money we demand. Certainly, given two equally risky projects that provide similar health benefits to the community, we would always choose to undertake one with a greater anticipated return. More often than not, however, our situation revolves around whether the return on a specific investment is great enough to justify the risk involved.

Consider keeping funds in a passbook account insured by the Federal Deposit Insurance Corporation (FDIC). You might earn a profit or return (in nominal terms—we'll talk about inflation later) of about 2 percent. The return is low, but so is the risk. Alternatively, you could put your money in a non-

bank money market fund where the return might be considerably higher. However, the FDIC would not insure the investment and the risk is clearly greater. Or you could put your money into the stock market. In general, do we expect our stocks to do better or worse than a money market fund? Well, the risks inherent in the stock market are significantly higher than in a money market fund. If the expected return were not higher, would anyone invest in the stock market?

That does not mean that everyone will choose to accept the same level of risk. Some people keep all their money in bank accounts; others choose the most speculative of stocks. Some organizations are more willing than others to accept a high risk to achieve a high potential profit. The key here is that in numerous business decisions, the organization is faced with a trade-off—risk versus return. Throughout this book, when decisions are considered, the question that will arise is, "Are the extra profits worth the risk?" It is, we hope, a question that you will be somewhat more comfortable answering before you have reached the end of this book.

As noted, profits are not the sole reason that health care organizations exist. Sometimes profits are just a means to an end, and not an end in itself at all. Health care organizations should always make decisions that keep their underlying mission in mind. Throughout this book, we provide many techniques that can be used to help you make the best financial decision, other things being equal. But we realize that other things are not always equal. If two projects yield the same health benefit, the one with greater profits or lower risk is usually the better choice. However, if the health care benefits are not equal, then managers need to factor that into their decision-making process. Sometimes you may decide that you

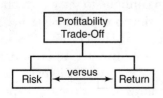

Figure 1-3 Profitability Trade-Off

are willing to accept a lesser profit or to take a bigger risk to hopefully achieve better health outcomes.

Viability

Health care organizations have no desire to go bankrupt, so it is no surprise that one of the crucial goals of financial management is ensuring financial viability. This goal is often measured in terms of *liquidity* and *solvency* (Figure 1-4).

Liquidity is a measure of the amount of resources an organization has that are cash or are convertible to cash in the near term to meet the obligations the organization has that are coming due in the near term. Accountants use *near term, short term,* and *current* interchangeably. Generally the near-term means 1 year or less. Thus, an organization is liquid if it has enough near-term resources to meet its near-term obligations as they become due for payment.

Solvency is the same concept from a long-term perspective, where *long term* means more than 1 year. Will the organization have enough cash generation potential over the next 3, 5, and 10 years to meet the major cash needs that will occur over those periods? An organization must plan for adequate solvency well in advance because the potentially large amounts of cash involved may take a long period to generate. The roots of liquidity crises that put organizations out of business often are buried in inadequate long-term solvency planning in earlier years.

So a good strategy is maximization of your organization's liquidity and solvency, right? No, wrong. Managers have a complex problem with respect to liquidity. Every dollar kept in liquid form (such as cash, T-bills or money market funds) is a dollar that could have been invested by the organization in some longer term, higher yielding project or investment. There is a trade-off in the area of viability and profitability. The more profitable the manager attempts to make the organization by keeping it fully invested, the lower the liquidity and the greater the possibility of a liquidity crisis and even bankruptcy. The more liquid the organization is kept, the lower the profits. This is essentially a special case of the trade-off between risk and return discussed earlier.

Similarly, there is a trade-off between providing health care services and viability. We cannot provide all the health care patients might want regardless of their ability to pay. Although providing charity care is often appropriate, there must be limits. If the organization decides to provide unlimited charity care without consideration of the financial implications, it may threaten its viability or continued existence.

Health care organizations have to temper their desire to provide health care services regardless of ability to pay with their desire to continue in business. It does not do the community any good for a health care provider to provide so much charity care in 1 year that it goes bankrupt and ceases operations. It is better for it to provide a measured amount of charity care so that it can remain viable. That way it can continue to serve the community, including the poor, on a long-term basis.

We mentioned that profitability and viability are not synonymous. An organization can be profitable every year of its existence, yet go bankrupt anyway. How can this happen? Frequently it is the result of rapid growth and

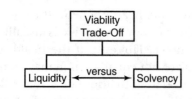

Figure 1-4 Viability

poor financial planning. Consider a privately held medical supplies company, Expanding Medical Supplies, whose sales are so good that it constantly needs to expand its inventory on hand. Such expansion requires cash payments to manufacturers well in advance of ultimate cash receipts from customers.

Assume that Expanding Medical Supplies starts the year with $40,000 in cash, $80,000 of receivables, and 10,000 units of inventory. *Receivables* are amounts its customers owe it for goods and services that they bought but which have not been paid for yet. Its inventory units (the medical supply items) are sold for $10 each and they have a cost of $8, yielding a profit of $2 on each unit sold. During January, it collects all of its receivables from the beginning of the year (no bad debts!), thus increasing available cash to $120,000. January sales are 10,000 units, up 2,000 from the 8,000 units sold in December.

Because of increased sales, Expanding Medical Supplies decides to expand inventory to 12,000 units. Of the $120,000 available, it spends $96,000 on replacement and expansion of inventory (12,000 units acquired at $8 each). No cash is collected yet for sales made in January. This leaves a January month-end cash balance of $24,000.

$	40,000	Cash, January 1
+	80,000	Collections during January
$	120,000	Cash available
−	96,000	Purchases of inventory
$	24,000	Cash balance, January 31

During February, all $100,000 of receivables from January's sales (10,000 units at $10 each) are collected, increasing the available cash to $124,000. In February, the entire 12,000 units on hand are sold and are replaced in stock with an expanded total inventory of 15,000 units.

$	24,000	Cash, January 31
+	100,000	Collections during February
$	124,000	Cash available
−	120,000	Purchases of inventory (15,000 units at $8 each)
$	4,000	Cash balance, February 28

Everyone at Expanding Medical Supplies is overjoyed. They are making $2 on each unit sold. They are collecting 100 percent of their sales on a timely basis. There appears to be unlimited growth potential for increasing sales and profits. The reader may suspect that we are going to pull the rug out from under Expanding Medical Supplies by having sales drop or customers stop paying. Not at all.

In March, Expanding Medical Supplies collects $120,000 from its February sales. This is added to the $4,000 cash balance from the end of February, for an available cash balance of $124,000 in March. During March, all 15,000 units in inventory are sold and inventory is replaced and expanded to 20,000 units. Times have never been better, except for one problem. Expanding Medical Supplies has only $124,000, but the bill for its March purchases is $160,000 (20,000 units at $8 each). It is $36,000 short in terms of cash needed to meet current needs. Depending on the attitude of its supplier and its banker, Expanding Medical Supplies may be bankrupt.

$	4,000	Cash, February 28
+	120,000	Collections during March
$	124,000	Cash available
−	160,000	Purchases of inventory
$	(36,000)	Cash balance, March 31

Two key factors make this kind of scenario common. The first is that growth implies outlay of substantial amounts of cash for the increased inventory levels needed to handle a growing sales volume. The second is that growth is often accompanied by an expansion of plant and equipment, again well in advance of the ultimate receipt of cash from customers.

Do growing organizations have to go bankrupt? Obviously not. But they do need to plan their liquidity and solvency along with their growth. The key is to focus on the long-term plans for cash. It is often said that banks prefer to lend to those who don't need the money. Certainly banks do not like to lend to organizations like Expanding Medical Supplies, who are desperate for the money. A more sensible approach for Expanding Medical Supplies than going to a bank in March would be to lay out a long-term plan for how much it expects to grow and what the cash needs are for that amount of growth. The money can then be obtained from the issuing of bonds and additional shares of stock (see Chapter 16), or orderly bank financing can be anticipated and approved well in advance.

Apparently, even in a profitable environment cash flow projections are a real concern. Liquidity and solvency are crucial to an organization's viability. Throughout the book, therefore, we return to this issue as well as that of profitability. In fact, the reader will become aware that a substantial amount of emphasis in financial accounting is placed on providing the user of financial information with indications of the organization's liquidity and solvency.

HOW DOES ACCOUNTING FIT INTO FINANCIAL MANAGEMENT?

As mentioned, accounting is like history with dollar signs. As with many things in life, we can learn a great deal from history. To that end, financial accounting (often taking the form of balance sheets and income statements) can help managers to make ongoing decisions to help the organization maintain both its prof-

itability and viability. In Chapter 2, we introduce the reader to the financial environment of today's health care organizations. There are a number of unique aspects of health care that require a solid understanding before one can start to completely understand accounting and financial statements that are generated by accountants. Chapter 3 introduces the basic accounting concepts used within the broader framework of financial management.

KEY CONCEPTS

Financial management—Management of the finances of the organization to maximize the organization's wealth and the achievement of its other goals.

Accounting—The provision of financial information.

a. *Financial accounting*—Provision of retrospective information regarding the financial position of the organization and the results of its operations.

b. *Managerial accounting*—Provision of prospective financial information for making improved managerial decisions.

Finance—Provision of analyses concerning the acquisition and disposition of the organization's resources.

Goals of Financial Management

a. *Profitability*—A trade-off always exists between maximization of expected profits and the acceptable level of risk. Undertaking greater risk requires greater anticipated returns.

b. *Viability*—A trade-off always exists between viability and profitability. Greater liquidity results in more safety, but lower profits.

TEST YOUR KNOWLEDGE

See www.jbpub.com/catalog/0763726753/ supplements.htm.

CHAPTER 2

Financial Environment of Health Care Organizations

Health care is an enormous part of the US economy, representing 17% of all personal consumption expenditures annually.[1] It has many different components, many different types of providers, and many different types of organizations all playing an important part in the overall delivery of health care. Health care is provided by for-profit organizations, not-for-profit organizations, and governmental organizations; there are service providers, suppliers, and insurers. In the end, it is a very complex maze of different organizations with different definitions of success and some differences in their accounting procedures and financial management techniques. This chapter highlights some of the most significant differences and issues within the financial environment of today's health care system.

HOW DO WE GET PAID?

Anyone who works in a health care organization knows that getting paid for services provided is never easy. The health care financing (or reimbursement) system is one of the most complex systems around. Unlike most industries, health care service providers are often paid by third parties. By *third party* we mean someone other than the individual receiving the medical care. This includes insurance companies, government programs, and other third-party payers. The patient is often caught in the middle of the maze of payment and insurance issues that plague the current health care system.

Although we cannot describe "the" payment system (because there are literally hundreds of payment systems), we can describe the basic flow of the money in today's health care payment maze. From the health care provider's point of view, the payment system starts with the delivery of service to a patient and the generation of a bill (a formal claim on cash). Most health care providers have established rates for different services called *charges*. In addition, however, providers also have rates that they have negotiated and agreed to with insurance companies as well as rates they must agree to accept from the government (mostly Medicare and Medicaid) if they choose to participate in those government programs. The difference between the provider's charge and the negotiated rate is referred to as a *contractual allowance*.

---

[1] *Source:* Derived from *Economic Report of the President 2005*, Table B-16—Personal consumption expenditures, 1959–2004.

Depending on the type of insurance and the specific insurance company, the patient may pay some portion of the bill at the time of the service (a *co-pay*), but generally either the majority of the bill or the entire bill is submitted to the insurance company for payment at a later date. The insurance company adjusts the charges on the bill for the contractual allowance and pays its share. Often the patient is responsible for either a deductible (e.g., the patient may have to pay the first $250 of incurred costs each year) or a co-pay (e.g., the patient may be responsible for 20% of the total cost of care after adjustment for contractual allowances). The payment cycle is completed when the provider receives the negotiated rate, which is usually a minimum of 30 days from the date of service and is often much longer. This is an overly simplistic depiction of the payment system. There are many variations to this, but it suffices for our purposes.

There are many different kinds of health care organizations. The payment system described is most applicable to health care provider organizations like physician practices, hospitals, clinics, physical therapy practices, and nursing homes. There are health care organizations that have a more traditional business model of payment, including medical equipment and supplies companies (supplying directly to the providers) and pharmaceutical companies. The more traditional payment model involves direct payment from the customer to the supplier (no third-party involvement).

WHY DO DIFFERENT PATIENTS PAY DIFFERENT AMOUNTS?

As described, many health care providers negotiate different rates with different insurance companies. In the obstetrics department of a hospital, for instance, there may be four women all delivering babies on the same day. All four women give birth via cesarean section with no complications. All four babies are happy and healthy. However, each woman's insurance company pays a different amount (Table 2-1).

As you can see, this is very confusing. Four patients all receive the same service, but each pays a different amount. It should also be noted that this is really a simplified

Table 2-1 Examples of Different Insurance Payments

	Patient One Medicaid	Patient Two Traditional Fee-For-Service	Patient Three Managed Care	Patient Four Private Payer
Hospital charge	$1,000	$1,000	$1,000	$1,000
Contractual allowance	$ 500	$ 100	$ 300	$ 0
Net charge	$ 500	$ 900	$ 700	$1,000
Patient co-pay	0%	20%	Often a flat amount	100%
Patient payment	$ 0	$ 180	$ 100	$1,000
Insurance payment	$ 500	$ 720	$ 600	$ 0
Total received by provider of care	$ 500	$ 900	$ 700	$1,000

version of what really may exist! Sometimes it makes you wonder how any health care provider ever gets paid.

Another problem is created by charity care. Some patients cannot afford to pay for their care and have no insurance. Many providers offer a sliding scale, allowing these patients to pay the amount they can afford. Often this is below cost. It is critical to make sure that the amount collected from the charity patients and the other patients is sufficient in total to cover all of the costs of all of the patients and also provide at least a minimally acceptable level of profits. Bad debts compound the charity care problem. Not all patients pay the amount of the obligation that they are responsible for. As if this all were not enough, insurers refuse to pay bills if there are significant errors. For example, if the patient ID number is incorrect, no insurance payment is collected. If the provider is unable to find the patient and get the correct ID after the claim has been rejected, they may never be paid for those services.

These differences in payment by different payers and the complexity of the different types of health care organizations all create issues for the financial accounting within health care organizations.

HOW DOES ALL THIS IMPACT FINANCIAL ACCOUNTING?

The most direct impact that the payment system has on financial accounting within the health care environment is that charges are not the same as revenues. Because most health care organizations have no expectation of getting paid full charges (they have negotiated discounts up front), the organization is not allowed to claim the full charge as revenue when it reports the financial results of its operations. Similarly, if you are giving away care for free, you cannot include the amount you would have charged for that care as revenue. On health care financial statements that show revenues and expenses, therefore, the first item listed is *net patient revenues,* which reflects the fact that contractual allowances and charity care are not included in the revenue amount. Health care accounting is therefore somewhat different from traditional accounting. Many of the differences can be traced to the unique manner in which health care organizations get paid and the unique manner in which the industry divides along for-profit and not-for-profit lines.

The unique nature of the health care industry does not change the basic premises and conventions of accounting (see Chapter 3). It does, however, require accountants and managers to be aware of the uniqueness of health care accounting. We therefore provide a broad overview at first and ultimately a more specific and thorough analysis of the intricacies of health care accounting. Where appropriate, we point out the many different ways a particular financial event can be portrayed within different types of health care organizations.

KEY CONCEPTS

Health care reimbursement system—The complex system of patients and insurers that pay (reimburse) for the care provided by the various health care providers.

Third-party payers—Insurance companies and governmental agencies that pay the majority of the cost of treating patients.

Contractual allowance—The difference between a provider's posted charge for service and the amount of payment agreed to by the provider and the third-party payer.

TEST YOUR KNOWLEDGE

See **www.jbpub.com/catalog/0763726753/ supplements.htm.**

CHAPTER 3

Accounting Concepts

In most MBA and MHA programs, an accounting course is required in the first semester of study. Accounting has frequently been referred to as the language of business. The buzzwords you encounter in accounting are used as a normal part of the everyday language of finance, marketing, and other areas of management. Receivables, payables, journal entries, ledgers, depreciation, equity, LIFO, and MACRS are a smattering of the terms that you encounter if you have any dealing with the financial officers of your organization. All these terms have their roots in accounting.

In Chapters 3 through 8, we focus on introducing the reader to accounting and to many of the terms used by accountants. Specifically, these chapters emphasize the financial accounting system, that is, reporting the financial history and current financial status of the organization.

BASICS

Accounting centers on the business entity. An *entity* is the unit for which we wish to account. Entities frequently exist within a larger entity. An entity can be a department, project, or organization. For example, Joe's Family Medical Office is an organization that is an entity. However, if it is not a corpo-

ration and Joe owns it solely, the Internal Revenue Service considers it to be part of the larger entity *Joe*. That larger entity includes Joe's salary, other investments, and various other sources of income in addition to the Family Medical Office.

From an accounting standpoint, there are two crucial aspects of the entity concept. First, once we have defined the entity we are interested in, we should not commingle the resources and obligations of the entity with those of other entities. If we are interested in Joe's Family Medical Office as an accounting entity, we must not confuse the cash that belongs to Joe's Family Medical Office with the other cash that Joe has.

Second, we should view all financial events from the entity's point of view. For example, consider that the Family Medical Office buys tongue depressors "on account." A transaction on account gives rise to an obligation or *account payable* on the part of the buyer and an *account receivable* on the part of the seller. For both the buyer and seller to keep their financial records, or "books," straight, each must record the event from their own viewpoint. They must determine whether they have a payable or a receivable.

We assume throughout this book that the organization you work for is the entity. Once we establish the entity we want to account for, we can begin to keep track of its financial events as they happen. There is a restriction, however, on the way in which we keep track of these events. We must use a monetary denominator for recording all financial events that affect the organization. Even if no cash is involved, we describe an event in terms of amounts of currency. In the United States, accounting revolves around dollars; elsewhere the local currency is used.

This restriction is an important one for purposes of communication. The financial accountant not only wants to keep track of what has happened to the organization, but also wants to be able to communicate the organization's history to others after it has happened. Conveying information about the financial position of the organization and the results of its operations would be cumbersome at best without this monetary restriction. Imagine trying to list and describe each building, machine, parcel of land, desk, chair, and so on owned by the organization. The financial statement would be hundreds if not thousands of pages long.

Yet, don't be too comfortable with the monetary restriction either, because currencies are not stable vis-à-vis one another, nor are they internally consistent over time. During periods of inflation or deflation, the assignment of a dollar value creates its own problems. For example, the values of inventory, buildings, and equipment constantly change as a result of inflation or deflation.

ASSETS

The general group of resources owned by the organization represents the organization's assets. An *asset* is anything with economic value that can somehow help the organization to provide health care to its patients, either directly or indirectly. The CAT scanner used in radiology is clearly an asset.

The desk in the chief executive's office is also an asset, however indirect it may be in treating patients.

Assets may be either tangible or intangible. *Tangible assets* have physical form and substance and are generally shown on the financial statements. *Intangible assets* have no physical form; they consist of such items as a good credit standing, skilled employees, and a reputation for high-quality care. It is difficult to precisely measure the value of intangible assets. As a result, accountants usually do not record these assets on the financial statements.

An exception to this rule occurs if the intangible asset has a clearly measurable value. For example, if we purchase that intangible from someone outside of the organization, the price we pay puts a reasonable minimum value on the asset. It may be worth more, but it cannot be worth less or we, as rational individuals, would not have paid as much as we did. Therefore, the accountant is willing to show the intangible on the financial statement for the amount we paid for it.

If you see a financial statement that includes an asset called *goodwill,* it is an indication that a merger has occurred at some time in the past. The organization paid more for the company it acquired than could be justified based on the market value of the specific tangible assets of the acquired organization. The only reason an organization would pay more than the tangible assets themselves are worth is because the organization being acquired has valuable intangible assets. Otherwise, the organization would have simply gone out and duplicated all of the specific tangible assets instead of buying the organization.

After the merger, the amount paid in excess of the market value of the specific tangible assets is called *goodwill.* It includes the good credit standing the organization has with suppliers, the reputation for quality and reliability with its patients, the skilled set of employees already working for the organization, and any other intangible benefits gained by buying an ongoing organization rather than by buying the physical assets and attempting to enter the market from scratch.

The implication of goodwill is that an organization may be worth substantially more than it is allowed to indicate on its own financial statements. Only if the organization is sold will the value of all of its intangibles be shown on a financial statement. Thus we should exercise care in evaluating how good financial statements are as an indication of the true value of the organization.

LIABILITIES

Liabilities, from *liable,* represent the obligations that an organization has to outside creditors. Although there generally is no one-on-one matching of specific assets with specific liabilities, the assets taken as a whole represent a pool of resources available to pay the organization's liabilities. The most common liabilities are money owed to suppliers, employees, financial institutions, bondholders, and in the case of for-profit health care organizations, the government (taxes).

OWNERS' EQUITY/NET ASSETS

Equity represents the value of the organization to its owners. It is the portion of the assets available to the owners of the organization after all liabilities have been paid. For an organization owned by an individual proprietor (a solo practitioner), we refer to this value as *owner's equity.* For a partnership (possibly a physician group) we speak of this value as *partners' equity.* For a corporation we talk of this value as *shareholders'* or *stockholders' equity.*

For not-for-profit health care organizations, we use *net assets,* given the lack of formal "ownership." *Net Assets* is used to describe the leftover balance when you subtract liabilities from assets. In this book we use the term *net assets* whenever the equity of the owners is meant. Except in the rare cases in which a topic is relevant only to not-for-profit health care organizations, the reader from a for-profit corporation, sole proprietorship, or partnership can simply convert the term in his or her mind to the appropriate one for their organization.

Net assets is often referred to as the "net worth" of the organization or its "total book value." In the case of a corporation, *book value per share* is simply the total book value divided by the number of shares of stock outstanding. It is important to keep in mind, however, that a share of stock may be worth a different amount than its book value for a number of reasons addressed in various places later in this book. For now, consider just one example—goodwill. If an organization develops a good reputation with patients and suppliers, that reputation helps it to generate future profits. But goodwill that you develop for your organization is an intangible asset that does not appear on your financial statements because accountants have trouble determining exactly how much goodwill you have, and what that goodwill is worth. Rather than take a guess at it, goodwill you develop yourself is simply ignored when financial statements are prepared. As a result, this unreported goodwill might result in the organization being more valuable than the amount reported on the books. But stock advisors (brokers) will estimate the value of that goodwill and take it into account in telling their customers the true value of the organization. Therefore, its stock price per share may exceed its book value per share of stock.

The net assets of an organization are quite similar to the equity (or ownership) that is commonly referred to with respect to home ownership. If you were to buy a house for $400,000 by putting down $80,000 of your own money and borrowing $320,000 from a bank, you would say that your equity (or ownership) in the $400,000 house was $80,000.

If the house were an outpatient surgery center owned by a large health care organization, the $400,000 purchase price could be viewed as the value of the outpatient surgery center asset, the $320,000 loan as the organization's liability to an outside creditor, and the $80,000 difference as the net assets, or the portion of the surgery center owned outright by the organization—its net assets.

THE ACCOUNTING EQUATION

The relationship among the assets, liabilities, and stockholders' equity is shown in the following equation and provides a framework for all of financial accounting.

$$Assets = Liabilities + Net\ Assets$$

The left side of this equation represents the organization's resources. The right side of the equation gives the sources of the resources. Another way to think about this equation is that the right side represents the claims on the resources: the liabilities represent the legal claims of the organization's creditors, and the net assets represent the organization's claim on any resources not needed to meet its liabilities.

This equation is true for any entity. Once the organization's assets and liabilities have been defined, the value of its net assets is merely a residual value. The organization or its owners own all of the value of the assets not needed to pay off obligations to creditors. Therefore, the equation need not ever

be imbalanced because there is effectively one term on the equation, *net assets,* that changes automatically to keep the equation in balance. We refer to this basic equation of accounting throughout this book.

FUND ACCOUNTING

Not-for-profit organizations, including many health care organizations, have a unique element of financial accounting referred to as *fund accounting.* A *fund* is an accounting entity with its own separate set of financial records. A single health care organization can have a number of different funds. That is, we can think of a large health care provider that is an entity. But that entity is made up of many smaller subentities.

The easiest example of a distinct fund within a health care organization is a development fund, which is often a separate accounting entity that exists solely to collect charitable gifts from donors. Donors are often concerned that the money they give be used in the manner they specified at the time of the gift. In most cases, gifts are not for general operations. The organization therefore creates a separate accounting entity called a fund to help ensure that the donors' funds are used in accordance with their wishes.

As a separate accounting entity, each fund tracks its financial transactions and records separately. At the end of the fiscal year, each fund may produce separate financial statements, although the organization must prepare one set of financial statements that contains information for all of the funds combined.

Fund accounting also brings with it yet another term for net assets. In this case, *net assets* is sometimes referred to as *fund balance.* In mathematical terms, the fund balance is simply the difference between assets and liabilities. If we took the funds assets and paid off the liabilities, the amount that would be left is the balance in the fund, or simply the fund balance. Remember, we now have a number of different terms that represent the same concept, but are used for different organizations, namely, *owner's equity, partners' equity, stockholders' equity, net assets,* and *fund balance.* Throughout this text, we predominantly use the term *net assets.*

GENERALLY ACCEPTED ACCOUNTING PRINCIPLES

Accounting is not a physical science like chemistry or biology; there are no laws of nature at work. In fact, accounting is more of an art than a science. If there are no laws of nature, then how do we know that different organizations are following the same rules with respect to how they account for their financial performance? One accountant (artist) could choose to account for (or paint) the history of his or her organization using one approach while another account-

ant across the street uses a different approach. In many instances, strong arguments can be posed for alternative accounting treatments. Selection of one uniform set of rules for all organizations is not, however, a simple exercise.

For example, consider a pharmaceutical company that is developing new drugs. Hypothetically, suppose that for every 20 drugs developed and put into clinical trials, the industry average is 1 drug becoming a commercially viable product.

The pharmaceutical company hypothetically expects to spend $100 million developing each new drug and expects to recover $20 billion worth of revenue from the one commercially viable drug. After 1 year, 10 drugs have been developed at a cost of $1 billion, and no commercially viable drug has been approved for sale. Consider how the company might present this on its financial statements. Table 3-1 provides income statements under three alternative accounting methods. (An *income,* or *operating, statement*

Table 3-1 Alternative Accounting Methods for New Drug Development

	Year One	Year Two	
	Actual Result	**If Drug Developed**	**If No Drug**
Method One			
Revenue	$ 0	$20,000,000,000	$ 0
Less Expense	1,000,000,000	1,000,000,000	1,000,000,000
Net Income	$(1,000,000,000)	$19,000,000,000	$ (1,000,000,000)
Method Two			
Revenue	$ 0	$20,000,000,000	$ 0
Less expense	0	2,000,000,000	2,000,000,000
Net Income	$ 0	$18,000,000,000	$ (2,000,000,000)
Method Three			
Revenue	$ 10,000,000,000	$10,000,000,000	$(10,000,000,000)
Less expense	1,000,000,000	1,000,000,000	1,000,000,000
Net Income	$ 9,000,000,000	$ 9,000,000,000	$(11,000,000,000)

is a financial statement that provides information on whether the organization has earned a profit or loss for the year, and if so, how much. We more formally introduce income statements in Chapter 4). As you look at Table 3-1, note that putting parentheses around a number is an accountant's indication of a negative number.

In all three methods, net income is the same for the 2-year period. If the pharmaceutical company develops a viable drug, it will receive $20 billion in return for a 2-year cost of $2 billion, leaving a profit of $18 billion. If the company doesn't discover a viable drug, then the combined 2 years must indicate an expenditure of $2 billion with no revenue, or a loss of $2 billion.

Although the 2-year totals are the same under all three methods, viable drug or no viable drug, the profit reported in each year varies substantially depending on the method chosen. Method one takes things as they come. In year one no viable drug is developed, so the $1 billion spent is all considered to be gone. The company reports a loss of $1 billion for the year.

Method two argues that the $1 billion was an investment in a 2-year project rather than being a loss. On the basis of the hypothetical pharmaceutical industry average, the company will likely develop a viable drug next year, and it gives an unduly harsh picture of the company's results to show it as a loss. This method records no revenue or expense for year one.

Method three argues that because the company expects to develop a viable drug, and because half of the work is completed by the end of year one, the company should report half of the profits by the end of year one. In this method, $10 billion of revenue is recorded in year one, even though no viable drug has yet been developed. If no drug is developed in year two, the year one

revenue must be eliminated by showing negative revenue in year two.

Comparing the three methods at the end of year one leaves the user of financial statements with the information that the company either lost $1 billion, or broke even, or made a profit of $9 billion during the year. For the second year, if a drug is successfully developed and approved, the profits will be $19 billion for method one, $18 billion for method two, and $9 billion for method three. If no drug is successfully developed, method one shows a loss of $1 billion, method two shows a loss of $2 billion, and method three shows a loss of $11 billion.

You may have a favorite among the three methods. Accountants do not allow use of method three. It is considered to be overly optimistic, because there is a reasonably good chance that there may well be no viable drug developed at all. In that case, reporting $9 billion of profit in the first year is clearly misleading.

Methods one and two, however, each have strong proponents and substantial theoretical support. Accountants frequently prefer a conservative approach, and method one provides it. On the other hand, accountants like to "match" expense with the revenue it causes to be generated. This preference supports method two. In this example, the supporters of method one have carried the day. Amounts spent currently researching drugs must be treated as expenses in the year the research is being done. We cannot defer recognition of that expense to a future period when a successful drug might be developed.

This particular example highlights a major controversy in accounting. It represents only one of a number of situations in which the accounting profession has difficulty selecting one consistent rule and saying that it should be applied across the board to all organizations in all situations. There is no true theory of accounting to resolve these dilemmas. The only way to achieve a logical order is by agreement on an arbitrary set of rules.

Comparison of different organizations would be simplified if the set of rules selected permitted very little leeway for the organization. However, politically, accountants have not always been able to accomplish this because selection of one method over another will usually help one set of organizations and hurt another set. In most instances organizations have no choice, but there are a substantial number of situations where alternative rules are allowed.

However, the organization can choose from only a relatively narrow set of alternative rules. Whenever the organization makes a choice, that choice must be explicitly stated somewhere in the financial statements.

Who makes the rules that organizations must follow in their accounting practices? There is a rule-making body called the Financial Accounting Standards Board (FASB). The pronouncements of this board carry the weight of competent authority, according to the American Institute of Certified Public Accountants (AICPA). The AICPA is a body much like the physicians' AMA and has substantial influence with its membership, so much influence that all CPAs look to it to specify the rules their clients must follow. If the CPA chooses not to follow one of the rules, he or she is subject to strong sanctions.

The FASB's (pronounced faz-B) rules are called *Generally Accepted Accounting Principles (GAAP)*. GAAP (pronounced gap) constitute a large number of pages of detailed technical rulings. Following are just a few of the most universally applicable rules. As we go through the book, additional rules relevant to the discussion will be noted.

Going Concern

In valuing an organization's assets, it is assumed that the organization will remain in business in the foreseeable future. If it appears that an organization may not remain a *going concern*, the auditor is required to indicate that in his or her report on the financial statements. The rationale is that if an organization does go bankrupt, its resources may be sold at forced auction. In that case, the resources may be sold for substantially less than their value as indicated on the organization's financial statements.

Conservatism

Conservatism requires that sufficient attention and consideration be given to the risks taken by the organization. In practice this results in asymmetrical accounting. There is a tendency to anticipate possible losses, but not to anticipate potential gains.

There has been considerable argument over whether this rule actually protects investors. There is the possibility that the organization's value will be understated as a result of the accountant's extreme efforts not to overstate its value. From an economic perspective, we could argue that one could lose as much by failing to invest in a good organization as by investing in a bad one.

Matching

To get a fair reflection of the results of operations for a specific period of time, we should attempt to put expenses into the same period as the revenues that caused them to be generated. This principle of matching provides the basis for depreciation. If we buy a machine with an expected 10-year life, can we charge the full amount paid for the machine as an expense in the year of purchase? No, because that would make the organization look like it had a bad first year followed by a number of very good years. The machine provides service for 10 years; it allows us to make and sell a product or service in each of the years. Therefore, its cost should be spread out into each of those years for which it has helped to generate revenue.

Sometimes these principles conflict. The conservatism principle lends support to using the first method in the earlier drug company example. However, the matching principle lends support to the second method. Some of the most difficult reporting problems faced by CPAs arise when several of the generally accepted accounting principles come into conflict.

Cost

The *cost* of an item is what was paid to acquire it, or the value of what was given up to get it.

Objective Evidence

This rule requires accountants to ensure that financial reports are based on such evidence as reasonable individuals could all agree on within relatively narrow bounds.

For example, if we bought a piece of property for $50,000 and we could produce a cancelled check and deed of conveyance showing that we paid $50,000 for the property, then reasonable people would probably agree that the property cost $50,000. Our cost information is based on objective evidence. Twenty years after the property is purchased, management calls in an appraiser who values the property at $500,000. The appraisal is considered to be subjective evidence. Different appraisers might vary substantially as to their estimate of the property's value. Three different appraisers

might well offer three widely different estimates for the same property.

In such a case, the rule of objective evidence requires the property to be valued on the financial statements based on the best available objective evidence. This is the cost—$50,000! Consider the implications of this for financial reporting. If you thought that financial statements give perfectly valid information about the organization, this should shake your confidence somewhat. Financial statements provide extremely limited representations of the organization. Without an understanding of generally accepted accounting principles (GAAP), the reader of a financial statement may well draw unwarranted conclusions.

Materiality

The principle of materiality requires the accountant to correct errors that are "material" in nature. *Material* means large or significant. Insignificant errors may be ignored. But how does one define significance? Is it $5? $500? $5,000,000? Significance depends substantially on the size and particular circumstances of the individual organization.

Rather than set absolute standards, accountants define materiality in terms of effects on the users of financial statements. If there exists a misstatement so significant that reasonable, prudent users of the financial statements would make a different decision than they would if they had been given the correct information, then the misstatement is material and requires correction.

Thus, if an investor can say, "Had I known that, I never would have bought the stock," or a banker can say, "I never would have lent the money to them if I had known the correct total assets of the organization," then we have a material misstatement. The implications of this are that accountants do not attempt to uncover and correct every single error that has occurred during the year. In fact, to do so would be prohibitively expensive. There is only an attempt to make sure errors that are material in nature are uncovered.

Consistency

In a world in which alternative accounting treatments frequently exist, users of financial statements can be seriously misled if an organization switches back and forth among alternative treatments. Therefore, if an organization has changed its accounting methods, the auditor must disclose the change in his or her report. A note must be included along with the statements to indicate the impact of the change.

Full Disclosure

Accountants, being a cautious lot, feel that perhaps there may be some relevant item that users of financial statements should be aware of, but for which no rule exists that explicitly requires disclosure. So, to protect against unforeseen situations that may arise, there is a catchall generally accepted accounting principle called *full disclosure,* which requires that if there is any other information that would be required for a fair representation of the results and financial position of an organization, then that information must be disclosed in a note to the financial statement.

KEY CONCEPTS

Entity—The unit for which we wish to account. This unit can be a person, department, project, division, or organization.

Fund accounting—A system of accounting found in not-for-profit and government organizations that uses separate accounting entities (funds), each with its own set of financial records and financial statements.

Fund balance—The difference between assets and liabilities. Another term for net assets or owner's equity.

Generally accepted accounting principles (GAAP)—A set of rules used as a basis for financial reporting. Some key GAAP:

a. *Going concern*—Financial statements are prepared based on the assumption that the organization will remain in business for the foreseeable future. If that is not likely to be the case, it must be disclosed.

b. *Conservatism*—In reporting the financial position of the organization, sufficient consideration should be given to the various risks the organization faces.

c. *Matching*—Expenses should be recorded in the same accounting period as the revenues that they were responsible for generating.

d. *Cost*—The value of what was given up to acquire the item.

e. *Objective evidence*—Financial reports should be based on such evidence as reasonable individuals could all agree upon within relatively narrow bounds.

f. *Materiality*—An error is material if any individual would make a different decision based on the incorrect information resulting from the error than if he or she possessed the correct information.

g. *Consistency*—To avoid misleading users of financial reports, organizations should generally use the same accounting methods from period to period.

h. *Full disclosure*—Financial reports should disclose any information needed to ensure that the reports are a fair presentation.

Monetary denominator—All resources are assigned values in a currency, such as dollars, to simplify communication of information regarding the organization's resources and obligations.

Assets—The resources owned by the organization.

a. *Tangible assets*—Assets having physical substance or form.

b. *Intangible assets*—Assets having no physical substance or form; result in substantial valuation difficulties.

Liabilities—Obligations of the organization to outside creditors.

Owners' equity—The value of the firm to its owners, as determined by the accounting system. This is the residual amount left over when liabilities are subtracted from assets.

Net assets—The residual amount left over when liabilities are subtracted from assets.

Fundamental equation of accounting—Assets = Liabilities + Net assets.

TEST YOUR KNOWLEDGE

See **www.jbpub.com/catalog/0763726753/supplements.htm.**

CHAPTER 4

Introduction to the Key Financial Statements

This chapter provides a brief introduction to the key financial statements contained in annual financial reports. We discuss the balance sheet (or statement of financial position), the income statement (or statement of operations), and the statement of cash flows. These statements are crucial to understanding the finances of an organization.

THE BALANCE SHEET—HOW MUCH DO WE HAVE AND WHAT DO WE OWE?

The statement of financial position, more commonly referred to as the balance sheet, indicates the financial position of an organization at a particular point in time. Basically, it illustrates the basic accounting equation (Assets = Liabilities + Net assets) on a specific date, that date being the end of the accounting period. The accounting period ends at the end of the organization's year. Most organizations also have interim accounting periods. These periods often are monthly for internal information purposes and quarterly for external reports.

By default, an organization ends its year at the end of the calendar year. Alternatively, an organization may pick a financial or "fiscal" year end different from that of the calendar year. The year-end that an organization chooses is generally influenced by a desire to make things as easy and inexpensive as possible. One factor in the decision is the organization's inventory cycle (this is especially true for medical equipment and supply companies). At year end, most health care organizations that have inventories have to physically count every unit. If your inventory has a seasonal low point, this makes a good year end because it takes less time and money to count the inventory than it would at other times during the year.

Another factor in the selection of a fiscal year is how busy your accounting and bookkeeping staff is. At the end of the fiscal year, many things have to be taken care of by both your internal accountants and your external auditor. For organizations that are required to have an independent audit, there are time-consuming questions and information demands by the CPA. Tax returns must be prepared. Reports to the Securities and Exchange Commission are required for publicly held companies.

Thus, if you can find a time when the accounting functions within the organization are at a slow point, it makes for a good fiscal year end. For example, many academic medical centers end their fiscal year on June 30 because this date gives them all of July and August to get things done before students return to campus for the Fall semester.

The basic components of a balance sheet are shown in Table 4-1, which uses the hypothetical Keepuwell Clinic as an example. The first asset subgroup is current assets, and the first liability subgroup is current liabilities. *Short term*, *near term*, and *current* are used interchangeably by accountants and usually refer to a period of time less than or equal to 1 year. Current assets generally are cash or will become cash within a year. Current liabilities are obligations that must be paid within a year. These items get prominent attention by being at the top of the balance sheet. Locating the current assets and current liabilities in this way ensures that the reader can quickly get some assessment of the liquidity of the organization.

Long-term (greater than a year) *assets* are broken into several groupings. *Fixed assets* represent the organization's property, plant, and equipment. Fixed assets are sometimes referred to as *capital facilities.* Investments are primarily securities purchased with the intent to hold onto them as a long-term investment. Securities purchased for short-term interest or appreciation are included in the current asset category and are referred to as mar-

ketable securities, rather than as investments. Intangibles, although frequently not included on the balance sheet, are shown with the assets when accounting rules allow their presentation on the financial statements.

In addition to current liabilities, the organization also typically has obligations that are due more than a year from the balance sheet date. Such liabilities are termed *long-term liabilities.*

In the case of a not-for-profit health care organization, the last item on the balance sheet is either the Fund Balance or Net Assets. This represents the portion of total assets owned outright by the organization. In other words, it is simply the difference between assets and liabilities.

On the balance sheet, net assets are further divided into three categories:

- Unrestricted net assets
- Temporarily restricted net assets
- Permanently restricted net assets

Restricted classifications are usually tied to donor requests and requirements for how the funds are to be used. Donations that come with no strings attached and profit generated

Table 4-1		Keepuwell Clinic Balance Sheet December 31, 20XX		
Assets		**Liabilities and Net Assets**		
Current assets	$ 5,000	Liabilities		
Fixed assets	10,000	Current liabilities		$ 3,000
Investments	3,000	Long-term liabilities		4,000
Intangibles	1,000	Total liabilities		$ 7,000
		Net assets		
		Unrestricted		$ 4,000
		Temporarily restricted		2,000
		Permanently restricted		6,000
		Total net assets		$12,000
Total assets	$19,000	Total liabilities and net assets		$19,000

from daily operations are recorded as unrestricted net assets.

In the case of a for-profit corporation, the final entry on the balance sheet becomes a bit more complicated. Stockholders' or owners' equity consists of *contributed capital* and *retained earnings*. *Contributed capital* (sometimes referred to as *paid-in capital*) represents the amounts that individuals have paid directly to the organization in exchange for shares of ownership such as common or preferred stock. *Retained earnings* are the portion of the income that the organization has earned over the years that has not been distributed to the owners in the form of dividends.

Retained earnings, net assets, and fund balance, like all items on the liabilities and equity side of the balance sheet, represent a claim on a portion of the assets and are not assets themselves. Net assets of $100,000 does not imply that somewhere the organization has $100,000 in cash readily available that could be used immediately (perhaps as a dividend in a publicly traded health care corporation). It is far more likely that, as the organization earned profits over the years, it invested those profits in plant and equipment to generate future profits. Net assets really represent the organization's (or owners in the for-profit sector) share of ownership of the plant and equipment and other assets rather than a secret stash of cash.

Excel Template

Template 1 provides an opportunity to prepare a simple balance sheet for your organization. The template is available on the Web at www.jbpub.com.

THE INCOME OR OPERATING STATEMENT—HOW MUCH DID WE MAKE?

The *income* or *operating statement* compares the organization's revenues to its expenses. *Revenues* are the monies an organization has received in exchange for the goods and services it has provided. *Expenses* are the costs incurred to generate revenues. Net income is the difference between revenues and expenses. The simplest form of an income statement appears in Table 4-2. Unlike the balance sheet, which is a photograph of the organization's financial position at a point in time, the income statement tells what happened to the organization over a period of time, such as a month or a year.

The income statement is frequently used as a vehicle for the presentation of changes in net assets from year to year. By showing the difference between revenues and expenses for the year, the income statement gives a clear picture of the organization's change in wealth (or net assets). As mentioned, it is this wealth (or change in net assets) that enables the organization to invest in such things as buildings or equipment.

Although we use *income statement* at times in this book, that is only an informal name for the statement that reports revenues and expenses for health care organizations. The technical term for this statement for most organizations in the health care industry is the *operating statement* or *statement of operations*. Often, for-profit organizations in many industries refer to this statement as the *income statement*, and most not-for-profit organizations refer to this statement as an *activity statement*. The accounting profession considered whether for-profit health care organizations were more like other for-profit organizations or more like not-for-profit health care organizations. And whether not-

Table 4-2	Keepuwell Clinic Operating Statement For the Year Ending December 31, 20XX
Revenues	$20,000
Less expenses	12,000
Net income	$ 8,000

for-profit health care organizations were more like other types of not-for-profit organizations or more like for-profit health care organizations. Ultimately, the decision was that, for the most part, health care organizations, at least health care providers, were pretty similar and should be treated as similarly to each other as possible. Rather than officially call this statement an income statement (and imply not-for-profit health care organizations are like for-profit organizations) or call it an activity statement (and imply for-profit health care organizations are like not-for-profit organizations), it was decided that all health care providers would use the term *operating statement* or *statement of operations* to report their revenues and expenses.

Excel Template

Template 2 provides an opportunity to prepare a simple operating statement for your organization. The template is available on the Web at www.jbpub.com.

STATEMENT OF CASH FLOWS— WHERE DID ALL OUR CASH GO?

The third major financial statement is the cash flow statement, which provides information about the organization's cash inflows and outflows. The current assets section of the balance sheet of the organization shows how much cash the organization has at the end of each accounting period. This can be compared from year to year to see how much the cash balance has changed. However, that gives little information about how or why it has changed.

Looking only at the balance sheet can result in erroneous interpretations of financial statement information. For example, an organization experiencing a liquidity crisis (inadequate cash to meet its currently due obligations) may sell off a profitable part of its business. The immediate cash injection

from the sale may result in a substantial cash balance at year end. On the balance sheet this may make the organization appear to be quite liquid and stable. However, selling off the profitable portion of the business may have pushed the organization even closer to bankruptcy. There is a need to explicitly show how the organization obtained that cash.

The *statement of cash flows* details where cash resources come from and how they are used. It provides more valuable information about liquidity than can be obtained from the balance sheet and income statements. Table 4-3 presents a simplified example of what a statement of cash flows would look like.

Excel Template

Template 3 provides an opportunity to prepare a cash flow statement for your organization. The template is available on the Web at www.jbpub.com.

Table 4-3   Keepuwell Clinic
Statement of Cash Flows
For the Year Ending December 31, 20XX

Cash flows from operating activities	
Collections	$19,000
Payments to suppliers	(8,000)
Payments to employees	(3,000)
Net cash from operating activities	$ 8,000
Cash flow from investing activities	
Purchase of new equipment	($6,000)
Net cash used for investing activities	($6,000)
Cash flow from financing activities	
Borrowing from creditors	$ 2,000
Debt payment	(1,000)
Net cash from financing activities	$ 1,000
Net increase/(decrease) in cash	$ 3,000
Cash, beginning of year	1,000
Cash, end of year	$ 4,000

NOTES TO FINANCIAL STATEMENTS—WHAT DO THE FINANCIAL STATEMENTS REALLY MEAN?

As you continue to read this book, you will find that the accounting numbers don't always tell the entire story. For a variety of reasons, financial statements tend to be inadequate to fully convey the results of operations and the financial position of the organization.

As a result, accountants require that notes be provided to supplement the financial statements discussed. These notes provide detailed explanations and are included in annual reports as an integral part of the overall financial statements (see Chapter 12).

KEY CONCEPTS

Fiscal year end—The organization's year end should occur at a slow point in the organization's normal activity to reduce disruption caused in determining the organi-zation's results of operations and year-end financial position.

The balance sheet—Tells the financial position of the organization at a point in time.

Asset classification—Assets are commonly classified on the balance sheet as current, fixed, investments, and intangibles.

Liability classification—Liabilities are generally divided into current and long-term categories.

Net assets—the portion of total assets not required to repay obligations owed to creditors.

a. *Unrestricted net assets* result from donations that are given without restrictions and from operating profits. They are available to use as the organization sees fit.

b. *Temporarily restricted net assets* have some time or use restriction imposed by a donor.

c. *Permanently restricted net assets* are assets with specific restrictions imposed by a donor that prevent them from ever being consumed. However, they may be invested, and the earnings on the investment can generally be used for operating purposes.

Stockholders' equity is divided into contributed capital and retained earnings.

a. *Contributed* or *paid-in capital* is the amount the organization has received in exchange for shares of stock that reflect ownership of the organization.

b. *Retained earnings* are the profits earned by the organization over its lifetime that have not been distributed to its owners in the form of dividends.

Income or operating statement—A summary of the organization's revenues and expenses for the accounting period (month, quarter, year).

Statement of cash flows—Shows the sources and uses of the organization's cash.

Notes to the financial statements—Vital information supplementing the key financial statements.

TEST YOUR KNOWLEDGE

See www.jbpub.com/catalog/0763726753/supplements.htm.

CHAPTER 5

Valuation of Assets and Equities

One would not expect there to be much controversy over the valuation of balance sheet items. Wouldn't they simply be recorded at what they're worth? Unfortunately, it isn't as easy as that. Consider having bought a car 3 years ago for $25,000. Today it might cost you $28,000 to buy a similar car. Is your car worth $25,000 or $28,000?

Wait, it's more complicated than that. Your old car is no longer new and so its value has gone down with age. Because the car is 3 years old, and generally cars are expected to have a 5-year useful life, your car has lost 60% of its value, so it's only worth $10,000. However, because of inflation, you could sell the car for $15,000 and you'd have to pay $18,000 to buy it on a used car lot.

What is the value of your car? Is it $25,000, $28,000, $10,000, $15,000, or $18,000? Obviously valuation is a complex issue. This chapter looks at how accountants value assets, liabilities, and stockholders' equity for inclusion in financial statements. In addition, several other valuation methods that are not allowed for financial statement reporting are discussed because they are useful to managers.

ASSET VALUATION—HOW DOES THAT OLD BUILDING SHOW UP ON THE BALANCE SHEET?

Historical or Acquisition Cost

Financial statements generally value assets based on their historical or acquisition cost. This is done to achieve a valuation based on the Generally Accepted Accounting Principle (GAAP) of objective evidence. If the organization values all of its assets based on what was paid for them at the time it acquired them, there can be no question as to the objectivity of the valuation.

For example, let's suppose that some number of years ago a hospital bought land at a cost of $10 per acre. Suppose that 1,000 acres of that land runs through the downtown area of a major city. Today, many years after the acquisition, the organization has to determine the value at which it wishes to show that land on its current financial statements. The historical cost of the land is $10,000 ($10 per acre multiplied by 1,000 acres). By *historical cost*, we mean the historical cost to the organization as an entity. The organization may have bought the land from previous owners who paid $1 per acre. Their historical cost was $1 per acre, but to our entity the historical or acquisition cost is $10 per acre.

Accountants are comfortable with their objective evidence. If the land cost $10,000 and the organization says it cost $10,000, then everyone gets a fair picture of what the land cost. However, one might well get the impression from the balance sheet that the property is currently worth only $10,000.

In fact, today that land might be worth $10,000,000 (or even $100,000,000). The strength of using the historical cost approach is that the information is objective and verifiable. However, the historical cost method also has the weakness of providing outdated information. It does not provide a clear impression of what assets are currently worth. Despite this serious weakness, historical or acquisition cost is the method that generally must be used on audited financial statements in order for them to be in compliance with GAAP.

For assets that wear out, such as buildings and equipment, the historical cost is adjusted each year to recognize the fact that the asset is being used up. Each year the asset value is reduced by an amount that is referred to as depreciation expense. Depreciation is discussed in Chapter 9.

Price-Level Adjusted Historical Cost

Accountants are ready to admit that the ravages of inflation have played a pretty important part in causing the value of assets to change substantially from their historical cost. The longer the time between the purchase of the asset and the current time, the more likely it is that a distortion exists between the current value of an item and its historical cost. One proposed solution to the problem is price-level adjusted historical cost (PLAHC, pronounced *plack*). This method is frequently referred to as *constant dollar valuation*.

The idea behind constant dollar valuation is that most of the change in the value of assets over time has been induced by price-level inflation. Thus, if we use a price index such as the Consumer Price Index (CPI) to adjust the value of all assets based on the general rate of inflation, we would report each asset at about its current worth. Although this approach may sound good, it has some serious flaws.

Unfortunately, not everything increases at the same rate of inflation. The land in the hospital example may have increased in value much faster than the general inflation rate. There is no easy way to adjust each asset for the specific impact that inflation had on that particular asset using price indexes such as the CPI.

Where does that leave us? Well, PLAHC gives an objective measurement of assets. However, it might allow an asset worth $10,000,000 to be shown on the balance sheet at only $110,000. Perhaps it is better to leave the item at its cost and inform everyone that it is the cost and is not adjusted for inflation, rather than to say that it has been adjusted for inflation when the adjustment may be a poor one.

Net Realizable Value

A third alternative for the valuation of assets is to measure them at what you could get if you were to sell them. This concept of valuation makes a fair amount of sense. If you were a potential creditor, be it banker or supplier, you might well wonder, "If this organization were to sell off all of its assets, would it be able to raise enough cash to pay off all of its creditors?"

Net is used in front of *realizable value* to indicate that we wish to find out how much we could realize net of any additional costs that would have to be incurred to sell the asset.

Thus, commissions, packing costs, and the like would be reductions in the amount we could expect to obtain.

This method doesn't seek to find the potential profit. We aren't interested in the comparison of what it cost to what we're selling it for. We simply want to know what we could get for it. In the case of the hospital's land, its net realizable value is $10,000,000 less any legal fees and commissions the hospital would have to pay to sell it.

Is this a useful method? Certainly. Does it give a current value for our assets? Definitely. Then why not use it on financial statements instead of historical cost? The big handicap of the net realizable value method is that it is based on someone's subjective estimate of what the asset could be sold for. There is no way to determine the actual value of each of the organization's assets unless they are sold. This always poses a problem from an accountant's point of view. Another problem occurs if an asset that is quite useful to the organization does not have a ready buyer. In that case, the future profits method that follows provides a more reasonable valuation.

Future Profits

The main reason an organization acquires most of its assets is to use them to produce the organization's goods and services. Therefore, a useful measure of their worth is the profits they will contribute to the organization in the future. This is especially important in the case where the assets are so specialized that there is no ready buyer. If the organization owns the patent on a particular process, the specialized machinery for the process may have no realizable value other than for scrap.

Does that mean that the specialized machinery is worthless? Perhaps, yes, from the standpoint of a creditor who wonders how much cash the organization could generate if needed to meet its obligations. From the standpoint of evaluating the organization as a going concern, a creditor may well be more interested in the ability the organization has to generate profits. Will the organization be more profitable because it has the machine than it would be without it?

Under this relatively sensible approach, an asset's value is set by the future profits the organization can expect to generate because it has the asset. However, the problem of dealing with subjective estimates arises once again. Here we are even worse off than with the previous valuation approach. At least we can get outside and hire independent appraisers to evaluate the realizable value of buildings and equipment. However, under this method, estimates of future profit streams require the expertise of the organization's own management. Even with that expertise and an honest attempt to determine the future profits, the estimates often turn out to be off by quite a bit.

Replacement Cost

The replacement cost approach is essentially the reverse of the net realizable value method. Rather than considering how much we could get for an asset were we to sell it, we consider how much it would cost us to replace that asset. Although this might seem to be a difference that splits hairs, it really is not.

Suppose that last year you could buy a unit of merchandise for $5 and resell it for $7. This year you can buy the unit for $6 and sell it for $8. You have one unit remaining that you bought last year. Today, its historical cost is $5, the amount you paid for it; its net realizable value is $8, the amount you can sell it for; and its replacement cost is $6, the amount you would have to pay to replace it in your inventory. Three different methods result in three different valuations.

Replacement cost (often referred to as *current cost*) is another example of a subjective valuation approach. Unless you actually go out and attempt to replace an asset, you cannot be absolutely sure what it would cost to do so. While there might be an active market for inventory, and you can determine exactly how much you would pay for another unit, that is often not the case for your buildings and equipment. It is very hard to determine what it would cost you to replace one of your buildings, exactly, if something happened to it.

Which Valuation Is Right?

Unfortunately, none of these methods (see Figure 5-1) is totally satisfactory for all information needs. Different problems require different valuations. The idea that there is a different appropriate valuation depending on the questions being asked may not seem to be quite right. Why not simply say what it's worth and be consistent?

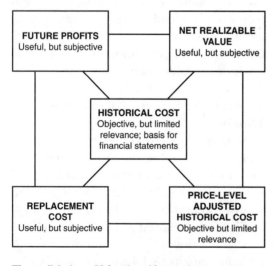

Figure 5-1 Asset Valuation Alternatives

From the standpoint of financial statements, we have little choice. GAAP requires the use of historical cost information and that restricts options substantially in providing financial statements. You might say, "Okay, the financial statements must follow a certain set of rules, but just among us managers, what is the asset's real value?" Still we respond, "Why do you want to know?" We really are not avoiding the questions. Let's consider a variety of possible examples.

First, assume that one of your duties is to make sure the organization has adequate fire insurance coverage. The policy is currently up for renewal and you have obtained a copy of your organization's annual report. According to the balance sheet, your organization has $40,000,000 of plant and equipment. You don't want to be caught in the cold, so you decide to insure it for the full $40 million. Nevertheless, you may well have inadequate insurance. The $40 million merely measures the historical cost of your plant and equipment.

Which valuation method is the most appropriate? In this case, the answer is replacement cost. If one of the buildings were to burn down, then our desire would be to have enough money to replace it. Other measures, such as net realizable value, are not relevant to this decision.

Suppose we are considering the acquisition of a new machine. What measure of valuation is most appropriate? We could value the machine at its historical cost—that is, the price we are about to pay for it. This method cannot possibly help us to decide if we should buy the asset or not. Looking at an asset's value from the point of view of its cost would lead us to believe that every possible asset should be bought, because by definition it would be worth the price we pay for it.

How about using the net realizable value? What would the net realizable value of the machine be the day after we purchase it? Probably less than the price we paid because it is now used equipment. In that case, we wouldn't ever buy the machine. How about using replacement cost? On the day we buy a machine, the replacement cost is the same as its historical cost.

Logically, why do we wish to buy the machine? Because we want to use it to make profits. The key factor in the decision to buy the machine is whether or not the future profits from the machine will be enough to more than cover its cost. So the appropriate valuation for the acquisition of an asset is the future profits it will generate.

Finally, consider the divestiture of a wholly owned subsidiary (perhaps a physician practice owned by a hospital) that has been sustaining losses and is projected to sustain losses into the foreseeable future. What is the least amount that we would accept in exchange for the subsidiary? Historical cost information is hopelessly outdated and cannot possibly provide an adequate answer to the question. Replacement cost information can't help us. The last thing in the world we want to do is go out and duplicate all of the assets of a losing venture. If we base our decision on future profits, we may wind up paying someone to take the division because we anticipate future losses, not profits.

The appropriate valuation in this case is net realizable value. Certainly we don't want to sell the entire subsidiary for less than we could get by auctioning off each individual asset.

As you can see, it is essential that you be flexible in the valuation of assets. As a manager, you must do more than simply refer to the financial statements. To determine the value of assets, you must first assess why the information is needed. Based on that assessment, you can determine which of the five methods discussed provides the most useful information for the specific decision to be made.

VALUATION OF LIABILITIES—WHAT DO WE REALLY OWE?

Valuation of liabilities does not cause nearly as many problems as valuation of assets. With liabilities, if you owe Charlie $50, it's not all that hard to determine exactly what your liability is; it's $50. In general, our liability is the amount we expect to pay in the future.

Suppose we purchase medical supplies at a price of $580 on open account with the net payment due in 30 days. We have to pay $580 when the account is due. Therefore, our liability is $580. The crucial aspects are that our obligation is to be paid in cash and it is to be paid within 1 year. Problems arise if either of these aspects does not hold.

For instance, suppose we borrow $7,000 from a bank today and have an obligation to pay $10,000 to the bank 3 years from today. Is our liability $10,000? No, it isn't. Banks charge interest for the use of their money. The interest accumulates as time passes. If we are to pay $10,000 3 years from now, that implies that $3,000 of interest will accumulate over that 3-year period. We don't owe the interest today, because we haven't yet had the use of the bank's money for the 3 years. As time passes, each day we owe the bank a little more of the $3,000 of interest. Today, however, we owe only $7,000, from both a legal and an accounting point of view.

You might argue that legally we owe the bank $10,000. That really isn't so, although the bank might like you to believe that it is. Let's suppose that you borrowed the money in the morning. That very same day, unfortunately, your rich aunt passes away. The state you live in happens to have rather fast processing of estates and around 1 o'clock in the afternoon you receive a large inheritance in cash. You run down to the bank and say that you don't need the money after all. Do you have to pay the bank $10,000?

If you did, your interest for one day would be $3,000 on a loan of $7,000. That is a rate of about 43% per day, or over 15,000% per year. Perhaps there would be an early payment penalty, but it would be much less than $3,000. Generally, accountants ignore possible prepayment penalties and record the liability at $7,000.

Another problem occurs if the liability is not going to be paid in cash. A health insurance company, for example, may receive advance payment for a year's worth of coverage. When it receives that money, it cannot record revenue right away, because it has not yet provided insurance coverage. Rather than revenue, when the insurance company receives the money it records a liability. What is it that the insurance company owes? The obligation is to provide financial coverage for health care needs that may arise over the year. We don't know exactly how much the payments will be, but we must make an attempt to value the liability. Take the example one step further and assume that the insurance company received $36,000 for the coverage, but hopes to only have to pay for $18,000 of health care. Is the liability $36,000 or $18,000?

In cases in which the obligation is nonmonetary in nature, we record the obligation as the amount received, not the cost of providing the nonmonetary item. What if for some reason the insurance company cannot provide the coverage? Will the customer be satisfied to receive a refund of $18,000 because that's all it would have cost the company? No, the customer needs to get the full $36,000 back, so the insurance company must show that amount as the liability. Over time, as the insurance company provides the coverage, they can reduce the liability in a pro rata fashion.

VALUATION OF NET ASSETS AND OWNER'S EQUITY—IS IT REALLY JUST WHAT'S LEFT OVER?

The valuation of net assets and owners' equity is relatively easy. Recall that assets are equal to liabilities plus net assets. Once the value of assets and liabilities has been determined, the net assets are whatever it must take to make the equation balance. Remember that net assets are, by definition, a residual of whatever is left after enough assets are set aside to cover liabilities. Thus, given the rigid financial statement valuation requirements for assets and liabilities, there is little room left for interpreting the value of net assets.

On the other hand, might there not be another way to determine the value of the organization to its owners? For a publicly held organization the answer is clearly yes. The market value of the organization's stock is a measure of what the stock market and the owners of the organization think it's worth. If we aggregate the market value of the organization's stock, we have a measure of the total value of the owners' equity.

Is the market value of the organization likely to equal the value assigned by the financial statements? Probably not. Financial statements tend to substantially undervalue a wide variety of assets; intangible assets that may be quite valuable are not always included in financial statements. Further, historical cost asset valuation causes the tangible assets to be understated in many cases. Thus, the organization's assets may be worth substantially more than the financial statements indicate. If the public can determine that to be the case (usually with the aid of the large number of financial analysts in the country), the market value of the stock will probably exceed the value of stockholders' equity indicated on the financial statements. Furthermore, stock prices are often dictated by the organization's ability to earn profits. In some cases, companies with few assets can still be quite profitable and therefore have a market value well in excess of the stockholders' equity shown on the balance sheet.

This discussion of valuation of assets and equities has left us in a position to better interpret the numbers that appear in financial statements. Financial statements are the end product of the collection of information regarding a large number of financial transactions. Each transaction is recorded individually into the financial history of the organization using the valuation principles of this chapter. Chapter 6 discusses the process of recording the individual transactions—how and why it's done. Chapter 7 demonstrates how all of the transactions, perhaps millions or even billions during the year, can be consolidated into three 1-page financial statements.

KEY CONCEPTS

Asset valuation—There are a variety of asset valuation methods. The appropriate value for an asset depends on the intended use of the asset valuation information.

a. *Historical cost*—The amount an entity paid to acquire an asset. This amount is the value used as a basis for tax returns and financial statements.

b. *Price-level adjusted historical cost*—Valuation method that adjusts the asset's historical cost based on the general rate of inflation.

c. *Net realizable value*—Valuation of an asset based on the amount we would receive if we sold it, net of any costs related to the sale.

d. *Future profits*—This valuation method requires each asset to be valued on the basis of the amount of additional profits that can be generated because we have the asset.

e. *Replacement cost*—Under this method each asset is valued at the amount it would cost to replace that asset.

Liability valuation—The value of liabilities depends on whether they are short term or long term and whether or not they are to be paid in cash.

a. *Short-term cash obligations*—Amounts to be paid in cash within 1 year are valued at the amount of the cash to be paid.

b. *Long-term cash obligations*—Amounts to be paid in cash more than 1 year in the future are valued at the amount to be paid, less the implicit interest included in that amount.

c. *Nonmonetary obligations*—Obligation to provide goods or services rather than cash, where the liability is generally valued at the amount received rather than the cost of providing that item.

Net assets and owner's equity valuation—Given a value for each of the assets and liabilities, net assets are the residual amount that makes the fundamental equation of accounting balance.

TEST YOUR KNOWLEDGE

See www.jbpub.com/catalog/0763726753/supplements.htm.

CHAPTER 6

Recording Financial Information

DOUBLE ENTRY AND THE ACCOUNTING EQUATION—THE GOLDEN RULE OF ACCOUNTING

Financial accounting consists largely of keeping the financial history of the organization. In performing financial accounting, the accountant attempts to keep close track of each event that has a financial impact on the organization. This is done to facilitate financial statement preparation. By keeping track of things as they happen, the accountant can periodically summarize the organization's financial position and the results of its operations.

To keep track of the organization's financial history, the accountant has chosen a very common historical device. In the navy one keeps a chronological history of a voyage by daily entries into a log. For a personal history, individuals make entries in their diaries. Explorers frequently record the events of their trip in a journal. Accountants follow in the tradition of the explorers, each day recording the day's events in a journal, often referred to as a *general journal*. The entries the accountant makes in the journal are simply called *journal entries*. The general journal is often called the *book of original entry*. This term is used because an event is first entered into the organization's official history via a journal entry.

In recording a journal entry, we need adequate information to describe an entire event. To be sure that all elements of a financial event (more commonly referred to as a *transaction*) are recorded, accountants use a system called *double-entry bookkeeping*. To understand double entry, we should think in terms of the basic equation of accounting. That equation is:

Assets (A) = Liabilities (L) + Net assets (NA)

Any event having a financial impact on the organization affects this equation because the equation summarizes the entire financial position of the organization. Furthermore, by definition this equation must always remain in balance. Absolutely nothing can happen (barring a mathematical miscalculation) that would cause this equation not to be in balance, because net assets has been defined in such a way that it is a residual value that brings the equation into balance.

If the equation must remain in balance, then a change of any one number in the equation must change at least one other

35

number. We have great latitude in which other number changes. For example, we might begin with the equation looking like:

A	=	L	+	NA
$300,000	=	$200,000	+	$100,000

If we were to borrow $40,000 from the bank, we would have more cash—assets would increase by $40,000—and we would owe money to the bank. Our liabilities would increase by $40,000. Now the equation would be:

A	=	L	+	NA
$340,000	=	$240,000	+	$100,000

The equation is in balance. Compare this equation to the previous one. Two numbers in the equation have changed. *Double entry* signifies that it is not possible to change one number in an equation without changing at least one other number.

However, the two numbers that change need not be on different sides of the equation. For example, what if we next bought some inventory for $30,000 and paid cash for it? Our asset "cash" has decreased while our asset "inventory" has increased. The equation now is:

A	=	L	+	NA
$340,000	=	$240,000	+	$100,000

The equation appears as if it hasn't changed at all. That's not quite true. The left side of the equation has both increased and decreased by $30,000. Although the totals on either side are the same, our journal entry would have recorded the specific parts of the double-entry change that took place on the left side of the equation.

DEBITS AND CREDITS: THE ACCOUNTANT'S SECRET

It wouldn't be much fun to be an accountant if you didn't have a few tricks and secrets. Later in this book we discuss a few of the more interesting tricks; for now you'll have to settle for a secret, the meaning of *debit* and *credit*.

Earlier an accountant's journal was compared to a navy logbook. That's not the only similarity. Sailors use the terms *port* and *starboard*. Many a time you've watched an old seafaring movie, and in the middle of a fierce storm, with the skies clouded and the winds blowing, the seas heaving and the rains pouring, someone yells out, "Hard to the port!" The sailor at the large oaken wheel, barely able to stand erect in the gusts of wind and the torrential downpour, struggles hard to turn the ship in the direction ordered. Perhaps you thought they were heading for the nearest port—ergo, "Hard to the port." Not at all. The shouted command was to make a left turn.

It seems that port simply stated means left and starboard really means right. Of course, it's more sophisticated than that; port means the left-hand side as you face toward the front of the boat or ship and starboard means the right-hand side as you face the front. Really what port means is debit, and starboard means credit. Certainly we can drape the terms *debit* and *credit* in vague definitions and esoteric uses, but essentially debit means left (as you face the accounting document in front of you) and credit means right.

Perhaps you had figured that out on your own, perhaps not. If you had, then you are potentially threatening to take away the jobs of your accountants and bookkeepers. To prevent that, some rather interesting abbreviations have been introduced to common accounting usage. Rarely will the accountant write out the words *debit* or *credit*. Instead, abbreviations are used. The word *credit* is abbreviated Cr. Got it? Then you can guess the abbreviation for debit: Dr. If you didn't guess it's not too surprising, given the absence of the letter "r" from the word debit. How did this abbreviation come about? Accounting as we know it today has its roots in Italy during the 1400s. Italy is the home of Latin, and were we to trace the word debit back to its Latin roots, the "r" would turn up.

Debit and *credit* deserve a little more clarification. Prior to actually using *debit* and *credit,* accountants perform a modification to the accounting equation (that is, Assets (A) equal Liabilities (L) plus Net Assets (NA)). Essentially, this modification requires examination of what causes net assets to change. As presented, the balance sheet equation is:

$$A = L + NA$$

To find out where we are at the end of a year, we need to know where we started and what changes occurred during the year. The changes in assets are equal to the change in liabilities plus the change in net assets, or:

$$\Delta A = \Delta L + \Delta NA$$

where the symbol "Δ" indicates a change in some number. For example, ΔA represents the change in assets.

Moving a step further, net assets increase as a result of revenues (R) and decrease as a result of expenses (E). Revenues make owners better off and expenses make owners worse off. Therefore, our basic equation of accounting now indicates that the change in assets is equal to the change in liabilities, plus the change in revenues less expenses, or in equation form:

$$\Delta A = \Delta L + \Delta R - \Delta E$$

The only problem with this equation as it now stands is that accountants are very fond of addition, but only tolerate subtraction when absolutely necessary. The above equation can be manipulated using algebra. We can add the change in expenses to both sides of the equation. Doing so produces the following equation:

$$\Delta A + \Delta E = \Delta L + \Delta R$$

Having made these changes in the basic equation, we can return to our discussion of debits and credits. When we say that the debit means left, we are saying that debits are increases in anything on the left side of this equation. When we say that credit means right, we are saying that credits increase anything on the right side of this equation. Of course, that leaves us with a slight problem. What do we do if something on either side decreases? We have to reverse our terminology. An account on the left is decreased by a credit and an account on the right is decreased by a debit.

Debits and credits are mechanical tools that aid bookkeepers. Debits and credits have no underlying theoretical or intuitive basis. In fact, the use of debits and credits as explained here may seem counterintuitive. Cash, which is an asset, is increased by a debit. Cash is decreased by a credit.

If you think about this, it may not quite tie in with the way you've been thinking about debits and credits until now. In fact, what we've said here may seem to be downright wrong. Most individuals who are not financial officers have relatively little need to use *debit* and *credit* in a business context. We come upon the terms much more often in their common lay usage.

Most of us have come into contact with the terms *debit* and *credit* primarily from such events as the receipt of a debit memo from the bank. Perhaps we have a checking account and we are charged 30 cents for each check we write. If we write twenty checks one month, we will receive a notice from the bank that it is debiting our account by $6. Something here doesn't tie in with the earlier discussion of debits and credits.

If a debit increases items on the left, and assets are on the left, our assets should increase with a debit. But when the bank debits our account, it takes money away from our account. The discrepancy results from the entity concept of accounting discussed in Chapter 3. Under the *entity concept*, each entity must view financial transactions from its own point of view. In other words, the organization shouldn't worry about the impact on its owners, managers, or customers; it should only consider the impact of a transaction on itself.

When the bank debits your account, it is not considering your cash balance at all! The bank is considering its own set of books. To the bank, you are considered a liability. You give the bank some money and it owes that amount of money to you. When the bank debits your account, it is saying that it is reducing an item on the right; the bank is reducing a liability. To you as an entity, there is a mirror image. Whereas the bank is reducing its liability, on your records you must reduce your cash. Such a reduction is a credit. Therefore, receipt of a debit memo from another organization would cause you to record a credit on your books or financial records.

Consider returning merchandise to a store. The store issues you a credit memo. From the store's point of view, it now owes you money for the returned item. The store's liability has risen so it has a credit. From your point of view, you have a receivable from that store; receivables are assets. Thus you have an increase in an asset, or a debit.

In other words, about the best way to insult your accountant is to call him or her a credit (that is, liability) to the organization! You'll have to reflect on this new way of thinking about debits and credits for a while if you're not accustomed to it, and if you wish to become fluent in the use of debits and credits. Unfortunately, because the items on one side of the equation increase with debits and the items on the other side decrease with debits, and vice versa for credits, it can take a while before it becomes second nature. Imagine a product manager trying to explain to an accountant that a new product is going to generate extra cash of $100,000. The accountant says, "Okay, debit cash $100,000," and the product manager says, "No, no I said it will *generate* $100,000, not use it!" Of course the accountant replies, "That's what I said, debit cash a hundred grand!"

If you still find debits and credits to be somewhat confusing, don't be overly concerned. Trying to look at things from a mirror image of what you've been used to all your life isn't easy. Fortunately, debits and credits are simply bookkeeping tools, and you don't need to use them extensively to understand the concepts of accounting and finance.

RECORDING THE FINANCIAL EVENTS

Now we are going to work through an example in which we actually record a series of transactions for a hypothetical health care organization, Healthy Hospital, for 2007. The purpose of this example is to give you a feel for the way that financial information is recorded, and to show the process by which millions of transactions occurring during a year can be summarized into several pages of financial statements. At the same time, we use the specific transactions in the example to highlight a number of accounting conventions, principles, and methods.

Table 6-1 presents the balance sheet for Healthy Hospital as of December 31, 2007. From this balance sheet, we can obtain information about assets, liabilities, and net assets for the beginning of 2008. Year-end closing balances from the balance sheet will be identical to opening balances for the following year. Our basic equation at the start of 2008 is as follows:

A		L		NA
	=		+	
$300,000	=	$134,000	+	$166,000

To examine financial events during the year, we are interested in the change in this equation. As explained, the change in the equation may be stated as follows:

$$\Delta A + \Delta E = \Delta L + \Delta R$$

Table 6-1	Healthy Hospital Balance Sheet As of December 31, 2007	
Assets		
Current assets		
Cash		$104,000
Accounts receivable		36,000
Inventory		40,000
Total current assets		$180,000
Fixed assets		
Plant and equipment		120,000
Total assets		$300,000
Liabilities		
Current liabilities		
Accounts payable		$ 34,000
Wages payable		20,000
Total current liabilities		$ 54,000
Long-term liabilities		
Mortgage payable		80,000
Total liabilities		$134,000
Net assets		
Unrestricted net assets		$146,000
Permanently restricted net assets		20,000
Total net assets		$166,000
Total liabilities & net assets		$300,000

Every financial event is a transaction that affects the basic equation of accounting. We keep track of whether or not each transaction complies with the rules of double entry by examining its effect on this equation. After a journal entry is recorded, placing an event into the financial history of the organization, this equation must be in balance or some error has been made.

The way that accountants actually record journal entries ensures that the equation remains in balance at all times. Each journal entry first lists all accounts that have a debit change, and then lists all accounts that have a credit change. The account names for accounts with a debit change are recorded in a column on the left and the account names for accounts with a credit change are recorded on a column indented slightly to the right. Similarly, the actual dollar amounts appear in two columns, with the debit column on the left of the credit column.

For example, suppose that we buy inventory and pay $12 cash for it. One asset, inventory, goes up by $12, and another asset, cash, goes down $12. In journal entry form this would appear as:

	Dr.	Cr.
Inventory	$12	
Cash		$12

To record purchase of inventory for cash.

Notice that *Inventory* appears to be somewhat to the left, and the dollar amount on that line appears in the Dr. column. As noted, an increase in an asset is a debit. *Cash* is indented to the right and the dollar amount on that line is on the Cr. column. A decrease in the asset, cash, is a credit. A brief explanation is often recorded for each journal entry. In this example the explanation is that the purpose of the journal entry was "To record purchase of inventory for cash."

The total of all numbers in the Dr. column must equal the total of all numbers in the Cr. column, or the fundamental equation of accounting is not in balance.

In the example that follows, we indicate the impact of each transaction on the fundamental equation of accounting and then show how it appears in journal entry form.

Healthy Hospital 2008 Financial Events

1. January 2. Purchased a 3-year fire insurance policy for $6,000. A check was mailed. The starting point for making a journal entry is to determine what has happened. In this case, we have $6,000 less cash than we used to and we have paid in advance for 3 years worth of insurance. Any item that we would like to keep track of is called an *account*, because we want to account for the amount of that item. Here, the balance in our cash account (an asset) has gone down, and our prepaid insurance (P/I) account (also an asset) has increased. This results in offsetting changes on the left side of the equation, so there is no net effect or change to the equation.

ΔA $+$ ΔE $=$ $\Delta L + \Delta R$

Cash - 6,000 $=$ No change
                             on right side

P/I + 6,000

	Dr.	Cr.
Prepaid Insurance	$6,000	
Cash		$6,000

2. January 18. The hospital mails a check to its supplier for $30,000 of the $34,000 it owed them at the end of last year. (Refer to Table 6-1 for the accounts payable (A/P) liability balance at the end of the previous year.) This requires a journal entry showing a decrease in the cash balance and a reduction in the A/P liability to our supplier.

ΔA $+ \Delta E = \Delta L$ $+ \Delta R$

Cash - 30,000 $=$ A/P - 30,000

	Dr.	Cr.
Accounts Payable	$30,000	
Cash		$30,000

Notice that when we look at the impact on the equation, both cash and accounts payable are negative numbers; each decreases by $30,000. In the journal entry format, negative signs are never needed or used. The decrease in cash is a credit, and appears as $30,000 in the credit column. The decrease in accounts payable results in a debit and appears in the debit column.

3. February 15. The hospital places an order with an equipment manufacturer for a new piece of machinery. The new machine costs $20,000 and delivery is expected early next year. A contract is signed by both Healthy Hospital and the equipment manufacturer. In this case there is no journal entry, even though there is a legally binding contract.

For there to be a journal entry, three requirements must be fulfilled. The first is that we know how much money is involved. In this case, we do know the exact amount of the contract. Second, we must know when the transaction is to be fulfilled. Here, we know that delivery will take place early the following year. Finally, the accountant requires that there must have been some exchange and that the transaction be recorded only to the extent that there has been an exchange. From an accounting point of view, Healthy Hospital has not yet paid anything nor has it received anything. There is no need to record this into the financial history of the organization via the formal process of a journal entry.

This doesn't mean that the item must be totally ignored. If an unfilled contract involves an amount that is material, then the principle of full disclosure requires that a note to our financial statements disclose this future commitment. However, the balance sheet itself may not show the machine as an asset or show a liability to pay for it.

4. March 3. Healthy Hospital purchases inventory on account for $30,000. Healthy will use this inventory in the delivery of care for which they will be paid $60,000. The effect of this transaction is to increase the amount of inventory (Inv.) asset that we have and to increase a liability, A/P. Do we record the newly purchased inventory at $30,000 or the amount we will ultimately get paid? According to the cost principle, we must value inventory at what it cost even though it will be used to generate revenues that are greater than that amount.

$$\Delta A \qquad + \Delta E = \Delta L \qquad + \Delta R$$
$$\text{Inv} + 30,000 \qquad = \text{A/P} + 30,000$$

	Dr.	Cr.
Inventory	$30,000	
Accounts Payable		$30,000

5. April 16. Cash of $28,000 is received from third-party payers for services provided to patients last year. This increases one asset, cash, and reduces another asset, accounts receivables (A/R).

$$\Delta A \qquad + \Delta E = \Delta L + \Delta R$$
$$\text{Cash} + 28,000 \qquad = \text{No change}$$
$$\qquad\qquad\qquad \text{on right side}$$
$$\text{A/R} - 28,000$$

	Dr.	Cr.
Cash	$28,000	
Accounts Receivable		$28,000

6. May 3. Healthy Hospital treats and discharges a patient for which they used $58,000 worth of inventory and have billed the patient's insurance company the agreed-upon rate of $112,000. This is an income-generating activity. Healthy has revenues of $112,000 from the service. It also has an expense of $58,000, the cost of inventory used during treatment. (There would obviously be other costs directly related to treatment such as wages, but we will keep it simple for now.) We can treat this as two transactions. The first transaction relates to the revenue and the second to the expense.

First, we have generated patient service revenue (PSR) of $112,000, so we have to record revenue of $112,000. We haven't been paid yet, so we have an account receivable of $112,000. This leaves the accounting equation in balance.

The second transaction concerns inventory and expense. To provide the service, we used some of our inventory. Thus, we have less inventory on hand. This reduction in inventory is offset in the accounting equation by a corresponding inventory expense. Once again, this transaction leaves the accounting equation in balance.

ΔA	$+ \Delta E$	$= \Delta L +$	ΔR
A/R		=	Patient
+ 112,000			Services
			Revenue
			+ 112,000

Inv.	Inv. Exp.
- 56,000	+ 56,000

	Dr.	Cr.
Accounts Receivable	$112,000	
Inventory Expense	56,000	
Inventory		$56,000
PSR		112,000

7. June 27. Healthy Hospital places an $18,000 order to resupply its inventory. The

goods have not yet been received. In this case there is no formal journal entry. Our purchasing department undoubtedly keeps track of open purchase orders. However, as in the case of the equipment contract discussed earlier, there is no journal entry until there is an exchange by at least one party to the transaction. We haven't paid for the goods and the supplies have not yet been received.

8. November 14. Employees were paid $36,000. This payment included all balances outstanding from the previous year. Because we are paying $36,000, cash decreases by $36,000. Is this all an expense of the current year? No. We owed employees $20,000 from work done during the previous year. Thus, only $16,000 is an expense of the current year. Our journal entry shows that labor expense (Labor) rises by $16,000 and that wages payable (W/P) decline by $20,000. Note that three accounts have changed. Double-entry accounting requires that at least two accounts change. The equation would not be in balance if only one account changed. However, it is perfectly possible for more than two accounts to change. Here we can see that although three accounts have changed, in net, the equation is in balance.

$$\Delta A \qquad + \Delta E \qquad = \Delta L \qquad + \Delta R$$
$$\text{Cash} - 36{,}000 \quad \text{Labor} + 16{,}000 \quad = \text{W/P} - 20{,}000$$

	Dr.	Cr.
Labor Expense	$16,000	
Wages Payable	20,000	
Cash		$36,000

9. December 31. At year end, Healthy Hospital makes its annual mortgage payment of $20,000. The payment reduces the mortgage balance by $8,000. It doesn't seem correct to pay $20,000 on a liability but only reduce the obligation by $8,000. Actually,

mortgage payments are not merely repayment of a debt. They also include interest that is owed on the debt. If Healthy Hospital is making mortgage payments on its plant and equipment just once a year, then this payment includes interest on the $80,000 balance outstanding at the end of last year (see Table 6-1).

If the mortgage is at a 15% annual interest rate, then we owe $12,000 of interest for the use of the $80,000 over the last year (15% x $80,000 = $12,000). Thus, the transaction lowers cash by $20,000, but increases interest expense (IE) (also on the left side of the equation) by $12,000. The reduction of $8,000 on the right side to reduce the mortgage payable (M/P) account leaves the equation exactly in balance.

$$\Delta A \qquad + \Delta E \qquad = \Delta L \qquad + \Delta R$$
$$\text{Cash} - 20{,}000 \quad \text{IE} + 12{,}000 \quad = \text{M/P} - 8{,}000$$

	Dr.	Cr.
Interest Expense	$12,000	
Mortgage Payable	8,000	
Cash		$20,000

10. December 31. At year end, Healthy Hospital makes an adjustment to its books to indicate that 1 year's worth of prepaid insurance has been used up. Many financial events happen at a specific moment in time. In those cases, we simply record the event when it happens. Some events, however, happen over a period of time. Technically one could argue that a little insurance coverage was used up each and every day, so the accountant should have recorded the expiration of part of the policy each day, or for that matter, each minute.

There is no need for that degree of accuracy. The accountant merely wants to make sure that the books are up to date prior to issuing any financial reports based on them. Therefore, a number of adjusting entries are made at the end of the accounting period.

One might ask why the accountant bothers to make such an entry even then. Why not wait until the insurance is completely expired? The matching principle would not allow that. In each case of an adjusting entry, the overriding goal is to place expenses into the correct period—the period in which revenues were generated as a result of those expenses.

In the case of the insurance, we have used up one third of the $6,000, 3-year policy, so we must reduce our asset, prepaid insurance (P/I), by $2,000, and increase our insurance expense (Ins.) account by $2,000.

ΔA $\quad\quad + \Delta E$ $\quad\quad = \Delta L + \Delta R$

P/I - 2,000 $\quad$ Ins. + 2,000 $\quad$ = No change on right side

	Dr.	Cr.
Insurance Expense	$2,000	
Prepaid Insurance		$2,000

11. December 31. Healthy Hospital also finds that it owes office employees $6,000 at the end of the year. These wages will not be paid until the following year. This requires an adjusting entry to accrue this year's labor expenses. The entry increases labor expense and, at the same time, increases the wages payable liability account.

ΔA $\quad + \Delta E$ $\quad\quad = \Delta L$ $\quad\quad + \Delta R$

$\quad$ Labor + 6,000 = W/P + 6,000

	Dr.	Cr.
Labor Expense	$6,000	
Wages Payable		$6,000

12. December 31. The plant and equipment that Healthy Hospital owns are now 1 year older. To get a proper matching of revenues for each period with the expenses incurred to generate those revenues, the cost of this plant and equipment was not charged to expense when it was acquired. Instead we allocate some of the cost to each year in which the plant and equipment helps the organization to provide its goods and services. The journal entry increases an expense account called *depreciation expense* (Depr.) to show that some of the cost of the asset is becoming an expense in this period. In this year, the expense amounts to $12,000. The calculation of annual depreciation expense is discussed in Chapter 9.

The other impact (recall that the double-entry system requires at least two changes) is on the value of the plant and equipment (P&E). Because the plant and equipment are getting older, we must adjust their value downward by the amount of the depreciation.

ΔA $\quad\quad + \Delta E$ $\quad\quad = \Delta L + \Delta R$

P/E - 12,000 $\quad$ Depr. + 12,000 = No change on right side

	Dr.	Cr.
Depreciation Expense	$12,000	
Plant and Equipment		$12,000

These transactions for Healthy Hospital give a highly consolidated view of the thousands, millions, or quite possibly billions of transactions that are recorded annually by an organization. These few transactions cannot hope to have captured every individual transaction or type of transaction that occurs in your particular organization. However, in this brief glance, you can begin to understand that there is a systematic approach for gathering the raw bits of data that make up the financial history of the organization.

There may be an enormous number of individual journal entries for an organization during the year. Chapter 7 examines how we can consolidate and summarize these numerous individual journal entries to provide useful summarized information to interested users of financial statements.

T-ACCOUNTS

Accountants frequently use a device called *T-accounts* as a form of shorthand when they are considering the financial impact of transactions. For any account that might be affected by a transaction, the accountant draws a large T, and places the name of the account on the top. For example, in the first transaction for Healthy Hospital in 2008, Healthy purchased an insurance policy for $6,000. This affects both prepaid insurance and cash, and T-accounts would be set up as follows:

Cash	Prepaid Insurance

Within the T-account, any entries on the left side of the vertical line are debits, and any entries on the right side are credits. The purchase of $6,000 of insurance on January 2, 2008, generates a debit to prepaid insurance and a credit to cash as follows:

Cash		
	1/2/08	$6,000

Prepaid Insurance		
1/2/08	$6,000	

Often, T-accounts are used to assess the balance that remains in an account after a transaction. From Table 6-1, we see that at the end of 2007, Healthy had $104,000 in cash, and no prepaid insurance. We can add this information to the T-accounts, and then summarize the position immediately following the transaction to purchase the insurance as follows:

Cash			
12/31/07	$104,000		
		1/2/08	$6,000
Ending Bal.	$ 98,000		

Prepaid Insurance		
12/31/07	$ 0	
1/2/08	6,000	
Ending Bal.	$ 6,000	

Notice that when the beginning debit balance of $104,000 of cash is combined with the $6,000 credit transaction on January 2, the result is a $98,000 debit balance. The $6,000 credit reduces the total amount of the debit balance, in the same way that a negative number offsets a positive number.

The use of T-accounts by accountants for informal discussions and analyses is quite common, even though T-accounts are not generally part of the organization's formal accounting system. The biggest problem T-accounts create for nonaccountants is that negative signs are not used. Each part of a transaction, or journal entry, is recorded in a T-account on the left or right side of the T, depending on whether it is a debit or credit, respectively. When you look at a T-account, to understand if the account balance is increasing or decreasing as a result of a specific entry, the user needs to be aware of whether each specific account is one that increases with a debit or a credit. Simply keep in mind that assets and expenses increase with debits and decrease with credits. Liabilities and revenues increase with credits and decrease with debits.

CHART OF ACCOUNTS

Up to this point we have always referred to accounts by their names, such as accounts receivable or wages payable. In practice, most organizations find it helpful to assign code numbers to each account. This facilitates the process of recording journal entries in the computer systems widely used for accounting.

Typically, an organization uses a fairly systematic approach to assigning numbers. All asset code numbers must begin with 1, liabilities with a 2, revenues with a 3, and expenses with a 4, for example. A second and third digit provide more specific information. For example, cash might be represented by 100 and accounts receivable might be represented by 110. Most organizations have receivables from many customers. A second set of numbers might provide that detailed information. For example, 110-12850 might refer to accounts receivable from customer number 12850. The organization might therefore sell $5,000 of its product to customer 12850 on account. It would record a $5,000 increase in its account number 110-12850.

Charts of accounts can be quite flexible. If an organization has five divisions, it can set aside one digit for each division. That digit might come at the beginning or end of the entire account code used for each transaction. Also, the organization may choose to use the chart to identify specific programs, projects, departments, or other information. Thus, an account number might look something like 4-110-12850-028. This might indicate that the home health division (division 4 of the company's five divisions) has an account receivable (110) from customer 12850 related to hospice services (028).

Although this may appear to be complicated, it actually keeps things clear and simple once you know how the organization's chart of accounts is set up. The official chart of accounts provides the guide to the system of accounts used by any organization. It first defines the intended purpose of each digit and the meaning of each number contained in each digit. So the first thing you learn is that the first digit represents the division of the organization and that the specific number associated with each of the five divisions is listed. Next you learn the meaning of the second digit, which in this case indicates whether we are looking at an asset, liability, revenue, or expense. If the second digit is 1 in this system, it means we are looking at an asset. The next two digits indicate the specific asset, liability, revenue, or expense. Thus, the 110 after the first hyphen tells us that we are looking at an asset, specifically accounts receivable. And so on.

Generally, in addition to defining the meaning of each digit and providing all data needed to interpret an account number, a complete chart is also maintained. This allows a user to look up any specific account number. Bear in mind, however, that the chart of accounts is a dynamic document. New accounts are frequently added to an accounting system and it is important to keep the chart of accounts up to date.

KEY CONCEPTS

Double-entry accounting—Each financial event affects the basic equation of accounting. For the equation to remain in balance, the event must affect at least two items in the equation; therefore, the "double" entry.

Journal—A book (or computer memory file) in which all financial events are recorded in chronological sequence.

Debits—Increases in assets and expenses; decreases in liabilities and revenues.

Credits—Increases in liabilities and revenues; decreases in assets and expenses.

Timing for recording transactions—Journal entries can be made only if we know with reasonable certainty the amount of money involved and the timing of the event, and if there has been exchange by at least one party to the transaction.

Adjusting entries—Most financial events occur at one specific point in time and are recorded as they occur. Some financial events occur continuously over time, such as the expiration of insurance or the accumulation of interest. Adjusting entries are made immediately prior to financial statement preparation to bring these accounts up to date.

TEST YOUR KNOWLEDGE

See www.jbpub.com/catalog/0763726753/supplements.htm.

CHAPTER 7

Reporting Financial Information: A Closer Look at the Financial Statements

Chapter 6 discusses how each of the numerous financial transactions affecting an organization can be recorded into the organization's financial history through the use of a journal and journal entries. When we get to the end of an accounting period (typically a month, quarter, or year), we want to report what has occurred. We need some method of summarizing the massive quantity of information we have recorded into a format concise enough to be useful to those who desire financial information about the organization.

Financial statements are used to present the organization's financial position and results of operations to interested users of financial information. As we learned in Chapter 4, financial statements are only several pages long. How can we process our journal entry information in such a way as to allow for such a substantial summarization? We do it via use of a ledger.

LEDGERS

A *ledger* is a book of accounts. An *account* is an item that we would like to keep track of. Every account that might be affected by a journal entry is individually accounted for in a ledger.

Although today many organizations have computerized their bookkeeping systems so that they no longer have a ledger book, you can think of a ledger as if it were simply a book. Each page in the ledger book represents one account. For instance, there is a page for the cash account, one for the inventory account, and one for patient revenue. Every time we make a journal entry, we are changing the amount that we have in at least two ledger accounts to keep the basic equation of accounting in balance.

An intermediate benefit of the ledger system is that it allows us to determine how much we have of any item at any point in time. For example, suppose that someone asked us on May 4th how much cash we currently have. One way to provide that information would be to review each and every journal entry that we made since the beginning of the year, determine which ones affected cash, and calculate by how much the cash total has changed. That presents an enormous amount of work.

Using a ledger approach, immediately after making a journal entry, we update our ledger for each account that had changed as a result of that entry. For example, in Chapter 6, the first thing that happened to Healthy Hospital in 2008 was a purchase of insurance for $6,000, which was paid for in cash. This expenditure requires us to go to the ledger account for cash and show a decrease of $6,000, as well as go to the ledger account for prepaid insurance and show an increase of $6,000. At the same time, we could update the balance in each account.

The ledger is, in some respects, a more complete picture of the organization than the journal is. Each year the journal indicates what happened or changed during that year. The ledger not only contains this year's events, but also tells us where we were when we started out at the beginning of the year. For instance, Healthy Hospital had $104,000 in cash at the end of 2007 according to Table 6-1. Our cash account in the ledger shows $104,000 as the opening balance at the beginning of 2008. Thus, when we purchased our insurance on January 2, 2008, we would be able to determine that our initial balance of $104,000 was decreased by $6,000, and that there is a remaining cash balance of $98,000. This gives a better overall picture of the organization than the $6,000 change alone does.

Essentially, the ledger combines account balances from the beginning of the year with the journal entries that were recorded during the year. All of the beginning balances for this year can be found by looking at last year's ending balance sheet. The balance sheet is the statement of financial position. The organization's financial position at the beginning of the year is identical to its financial position at the end of the previous year. Therefore, the ledger accounts start the year with balances from the year-end balance sheet of the previous year. During the year, the changes that occur and are recorded as journal entries are used to update the ledger accounts. The year-end balance in each account is the sum of the opening balance plus the changes recorded in that account during the year.

HEALTHY HOSPITAL'S FINANCIAL STATEMENTS

Table 7-1 presents the information from which we can prepare a set of financial statements for Healthy Hospital. This table represents a highly abbreviated ledger for the entire organization for the whole year. All of the journal entries for the year have been recorded. Each column represents one ledger account. That is, each column in this table is the same as one page in a ledger book. The opening balance is recorded for each account, based on information from Table 6-1, Healthy Hospital's December 31, 2007 Balance Sheet. The horizontal lines represent the individual numbered journal entries from Chapter 6. A running balance in each account has not been provided in this example.

A number of the ledger accounts in Table 7-1 start with a zero balance. This occurs for one of two reasons. The first reason is simply that there was no balance at the end of last year, so there is no balance at the beginning of this year. Such is the case with prepaid insurance. The second reason is that some items are kept track of year by year rather than cumulatively. The income or operating statement accounts relate specifically to the accounting period. We kept track of our income for 2007. Once 2007 was over and its results reported in our financial statements, we wished to keep track of 2008's income separately from 2007's. Therefore, all of the revenue and expense accounts start 2008 with a zero balance. When we get to the end of this year and ask "What was our revenue this year?", we want to know the revenue of this year separate and apart from any revenue we made in earlier years. The revenue and expense accounts are called *temporary accounts* because we start them over each year with a zero balance.

Table 7-1

Healthy Hospital
Ledger for 2008 (000's omitted)
Ledger Account

	Assets					+	Expenses					=	Liabilities			+	Net Assets			+ Revenue
	Cash	Prepaid Insurance	Accounts Receivable	Inventory	Plant & Equipment		Inventory	Labor	Interest	Insurance	Depreciation		Accounts Payable	Wages Payable	Mortgage Payable		Unrestricted	Temporarily Restricted	Permanently Restricted	Revenue
Beginning Balance	$104	$0	$36	$40	$120		$0	$0	$0	$0	$0		$34	$20	$80		$146	$0	$20	$0
1	-6	6																		
2	-30												-30							
3																				
4				30									30							
5	28		-28																	
6			112	-56			56													112
7																				
8	-36							16						-20						
9	-20								12						-8					
10		-2								2										
11								6						6						
12					-12						12									
Ending Balance	$40	$4	$120	$14	$108		$56	$22	$12	$2	$12		$34	$6	$72		$146	$0	$20	$112

The key to conveying financial information is the ending balance of each ledger account. As long as we are using a system in which each journal entry is *posted*, or recorded in the individual ledger accounts involved, we are able to determine the ending balance in each account. These ending balances provide the information needed to prepare a complete set of financial statements.

Excel Template

Use Template 4 to record journal entries, post them to ledger accounts, and calculate ending balances that can be used to prepare financial statements. This template is on the Web at www.jbpub.com.

The Operating Statement

Table 7-2 presents the 2008 Operating Statement for Healthy Hospital. The operating statement for any organization consists merely of a comparison of its revenues and expenses. To prepare this statement, we look at the ending balance in each revenue and expense ledger account. The ending balance in the revenue account at the bottom of Table 7-1 shows revenue of $112,000, which is exactly the same as the revenue in the operating statement in Table 7-2. You can compare each of the expenses between Tables 7-1 and 7-2 as well, and find them to be the same. This must be so, because the way that the operating statement was prepared was to simply take the ending balances from each of the revenue and expense ledger accounts.

Notice that the last line in Table 7-2 is called the *Increase in net assets*. For-profit health care organizations often refer to this as *Net income*, whereas not-for-profit organizations indicate either an *Increase in net assets* or a *Decrease in net assets*. If financial statements for 2 years are shown side by side, and there was a profit 1 year and a loss the other, the heading becomes *Change in net assets*.

Where did the "increase in net assets" terminology come from? Generally, all organizations, whether for-profit or not-for-profit, attempt to earn a profit each year. However, many not-for-profit organizations are uncomfortable subtracting expenses from revenue and reporting the difference as net income. They fear that would give the public an incorrect impression—the public might view the organization as a for-profit organization when they see that it has earned income. This could significantly reduce donations that the organization might hope to receive.

So an alternative name was sought for the difference between revenues and expenses. Revenue transactions result in an increase in net assets. For example, you provide care and get paid $100 for that care. Cash goes up $100 on the left side of the fundamental equation and revenue goes up $100 on the right side in the net assets category. So, net assets increase by $100. Suppose that it cost $80 to provide that care. Expenses result in either a decrease in assets or an increase in a liability, and also in a decrease in net assets. So, net assets would have declined by $80. Because net assets rose by $100 and declined by $80, there was a $20 change in net assets. Because it was a positive net change, it can be referred to as an *increase in net assets*.

Table 7-2	Healthy Hospital Operating Statement For the Year Ending December 31, 2008	
Revenue		$ 112,000
Less expenses		
Inventory	$ 56,000	
Labor	22,000	
Interest	12,000	
Insurance	2,000	
Depreciation	12,000	
Total expenses		104,000
Increase in net assets		$ 8,000

The Balance Sheet

The net assets ledger accounts (unrestricted, temporarily restricted, and permanently restricted) in Table 7-1 have the same balance at the end of the year as they had at the beginning of the year. As noted, the net assets of an organization increase when it has revenue and decrease when it has expense. In fact, every revenue increases net assets, and all expenses decrease it. We have had both revenues and expenses, but the net assets accounts have not changed. The reason for this is that we have simply been keeping track of the specific changes in revenues and expenses separately, instead of immediately showing their impact on the net asset accounts.

By keeping track of revenues and expenses in detail rather than directly indicating their impact on net assets, we have generated additional information. This information has been used to derive an operating statement. If we simply changed net assets directly whenever we had a revenue or expense, we would not have had the information needed to produce that statement.

Nevertheless, we cannot produce a balance sheet without updating the information in our net asset accounts. Table 7-3 provides a statement that updates all of the net asset accounts. In Table 7-3, we can see that both of the restricted net asset accounts did not change this year. Usually these accounts change as a result of gifts from donors. The increase in unrestricted net assets is a result of the difference between the $112,000 of revenues and the $104,000 of expenses.

All of the information used in Table 7-3 comes directly or indirectly from the ledger accounts shown in Table 7-1. The increase in net assets figure in Table 7-3 does not appear anywhere in Table 7-1. It is a summary of the year-end revenue and expense items from the operating statement (Table 7-2). All of the Table 7-2 items came directly from Table 7-1. We now have all of the information we need to produce a balance sheet.

The balance sheet for Healthy Hospital for 2008 appears in Table 7-4. The asset and liability balances came directly from Table 7-1 and the net asset balances came from our derivation in Table 7-3. The preparation of this financial statement is really quite simple, given the ledger account balances. The balances are transferred to the financial statement, with the main work involved being the determination of which accounts are short term and which accounts are long term.

Table 7-3	Healthy Hospital Analysis of Changes in Net Assets For the Year Ending December 31, 2008		
	Unrestricted Net Assets	**Temporarily Restricted Net Assets**	**Permanently Restricted Net Assets**
Beginning Balance 1/1/08	$146,000	$ 0	$20,000
Donor Gifts for 2008	0	0	0
Increase in Net Assets for 2008	8,000		
Ending Balance 12/31/08	$154,000	$ 0	$20,000

Excel Template

Template 5 uses the journal entry information from Template 4 to derive an Income Statement and Balance Sheet. The template is included on the Web at www.jbpub.com.

The Statement of Cash Flows

The one remaining financial statement that is widely used to report the results of operations is the statement of cash flows. As dis-

Table 7-4	Healthy Hospital Balance Sheet As of December 31, 2008	
ASSETS		
Current Assets:		
Cash	$ 40,000	
Prepaid Insurance	4,000	
Third-Party Receivables	120,000	
Inventory	14,000	
Total Current Assets	$ 178,000	
Fixed Assets:		
Plant and Equipment, net	108,000	
TOTAL ASSETS	$ 286,000	
LIABILITIES AND NET ASSETS		
Liabilities		
Current Liabilities:		
Accounts Payable	$ 34,000	
Wages Payable	6,000	
Total Current Liabilities	$ 40,000	
Long-Term Liabilities:		
Mortgage Payable	72,000	
TOTAL LIABILITIES	$ 112,000	
Net Assets		
Unrestricted Net Assets	$ 154,000	
Permanently restricted Net Assets	20,000	
TOTAL NET ASSETS	$ 174,000	
TOTAL LIABILITIES & NET ASSETS	$ 286,000	

cussed in Chapter 4, this statement focuses on the organization's sources and uses of cash. This statement also provides insight about the organization's liquidity, or its ability to meet its current obligations as they come due for payment.

The statement of cash flows shows where the organization got its cash and how it used it over the entire period covered by the financial statement. This feature is similar to the operating statement, which shows revenues and expenses for the entire accounting period, and is different from the balance sheet, which shows the organization's financial position at a single point in time. The statement of cash flows is divided into three major sections: cash from operating activities, cash from investing activities, and cash from financing activities.

The operating activities are those that relate to the ordinary revenue- and expense-producing activities of the organization. Organizations tend to be particularly interested in how their day-to-day revenues and expenses affect cash balances. These activities include items such as payments to employees and suppliers and collections of cash from customers. A controversial element involves interest and dividends. Many people believe that interest and dividends are more closely associated with investing and financing activities. However, interest and dividends *received* and interest *paid* must be included with operating activities because of their impact on revenues and expenses.

The investing activities of the organization relate to the purchase and sale of fixed assets and securities. It is clear that the purchase of stocks and bonds represents an investing activity. The accounting rule-making body determined that the purchase of property, plant, and equipment also represents an investment, and should be accounted for in this category.

Lending money (and receiving repayments) also represents an investing activity.

The financing activities of the organization are concerned with borrowing money (or repaying it), issuance of stock, and the payment of dividends. Note that when an organization lends money, it is investing. However, borrowing money relates to getting the financial resources the organization needs to operate. Thus, borrowing is included in the financing category, along with issuance of stock. For-profit organizations may choose to distribute some of their profits to their stockholders in the form of a *dividend*. Dividends paid are considered to be a financing activity because they are a return of financial resources to the organization's owners. They are not included in operating activities because dividends paid are not classified as an expense, but rather as a distribution to the organization's owners of income earned.

There are two different approaches to calculating and presenting the statement of cash flows. These are the direct and indirect methods. Table 7-5 presents an example of the Statement of Cash Flows prepared using the direct method. The direct method lists each individual type of account that resulted in a change in cash.

Looking at Table 7-1, we can see that cash was affected by transactions 1, 2, 5, 8, and 9. Review of each of those journal entries provides the information needed to prepare Table 7-5. For example, transaction 1 consisted of a $6,000 payment for insurance. Therefore, the decrease in cash was for an operating activity, specifically payment for insurance.

Table 7-5

Healthy Hospital
Statement of Cash Flows
For the Year Ending December 31, 2008

Cash flows from operating activities		
Collections from third-party payers	$ 28,000	
Payments to employees	(36,000)	
Payments to suppliers	(30,000)	
Payments for insurance	(6,000)	
Payments for interest	(12,000)	
Net cash used for operating activities		$ (56,000)
Cash flows from investing activities		
None		
Net cash used for investing activities		0
Cash flows from financing activities		
Payment of mortgage principal	$ (8,000)	
Net cash used for financing activities		(8,000)
NET INCREASE/(DECREASE) IN CASH		$ (64,000)
CASH, DECEMBER 31, 2007		104,000
CASH, DECEMBER 31, 2008		$ 40,000

This may be a cumbersome task when there are a large number of individual transactions. For example, how much cash was collected from customers during 2008? By looking at transaction 5 from Table 7-1, we know that the answer is $28,000. We can see the increase in cash and the reduction in accounts receivable. Typically, however, there are an extremely large number of individual journal entries related to receipts from customers.

Rather than review each transaction, accountants usually prepare the cash flow statement by making general inferences from the changes in the balances of various accounts. Note that accounts receivable at the beginning of the year were $36,000, and patient service revenue during the year was $112,000. Combining what was owed to us at the beginning of the year with the amount we billed patients and insurance companies this year indicates that there was a total of $148,000 that we would hope to eventually collect from insurers and patients. At the end of the year the accounts receivable balance was $120,000. Therefore we can infer that $28,000 must have been collected (the $148,000 total due us, less the $120,000 still due at the end of the year).

Let's consider another example. The mortgage payable account started with a balance of $80,000 and ended with a balance of $72,000 (see Table 7-1). Rather than reviewing all of the journal entries related to mortgage payments, accountants infer that $8,000 was spent on the financing activity of repaying debt. However, this inference process requires care. It is possible, for instance, that $40,000 was paid on the mortgage principal, but a new mortgage of $32,000 was taken on a new piece of equipment. The statement of cash flows must show both the source of cash from the new mortgage, as well as the payment of cash on the old mortgage. Therefore, preparation of

the statement requires at least some in-depth knowledge about changes in the accounts of the organization.

An alternative approach for developing and presenting the statement of cash flows is referred to as the *indirect method*. The indirect method starts with net income, or the change in net assets, as a measure of cash from operations. It then makes adjustments to the extent that net income is not a true measure of cash flow. Table 7-6 was prepared using the indirect method.

One of the most common adjustments to income is for depreciation. When buildings and equipment are purchased, there is a cash outflow. Each year, a portion of the cost of the buildings or equipment is charged as a depreciation expense. That expense lowers net income, but it does not require a cash outflow. Therefore, the amount of the depreciation expense is added back to net income to make net income more reflective of true cash flow. In Table 7-6 we see that the $12,000 depreciation expense is added to net income.

There are a variety of other items that cause net income to over- or understate the true cash flow. For example, if customers buy our product or service, but do not pay for it before the end of the year, then income overstates cash inflow. Therefore, in Table 7-6, there is a negative adjustment for the increase in accounts receivable.

Many of the adjustments to net income that are needed to determine cash flow from operating activities are quite complex. Therefore, many people prefer use of the direct method. However, because net income is considered essential to the process of generating cash, the net income reconciliation is required for cash flow statements to be considered to be in compliance with Generally Accepted Accounting Principles (GAAP). If the direct method is used, the Cash Flows from Operating Activities portion of the in-

Table 7-6	Healthy Hospital Statement of Cash Flows For the Year Ending December 31, 2008		
Cash flows from operating activities			
Net income			$ 8,000
Adjustments			
Depreciation expense		$ 12,000	
Decrease in inventory		26,000	
Increase in accounts receivable		(84,000)	
Increase in prepaid insurance		(4,000)	
Decreases in wages payable		(14,000)	
Total adjustments to net income			(64,000)
Net cash used for operating activities			$ (56,000)
Cash flows from investing activities			
None			
Net cash used for investing activities			0
Cash flows from financing activities			
Payment of mortgage principal		$ (8,000)	
Net cash used for financing activities			(8,000)
NET INCREASE/(DECREASE) IN CASH			$ (64,000)
CASH, DECEMBER 31, 2007			104,000
CASH, DECEMBER 31, 2008			$ 40,000

direct method (Table 7-6) must be included as a supporting schedule.

The information contained in the statement of cash flows is quite dramatic in this example. Although Table 7-2 indicated that there was a positive net income of $8,000, the organization is using substantially more cash than it is receiving. In some cases, this might reflect recent spending on buildings and equipment. A decline in cash is not necessarily bad. However, in this case, we note from the statement of cash flows (Table 7-5 or 7-6) that no money was used for investing activities. The largest decline in cash came from operations. What was the single largest

cause of the decline? Table 7-5 indicates that payments to employees were the largest item. They caused the largest cash outflow.

However, this is an example in which the net income reconciliation provides particularly useful information. Looking at the cash flows from the operating activities section of Table 7-6, the most striking number is the $84,000 increase in receivables. A growing company is likely to have growing receivables. In this case, however, the growth in receivables seems unusually large. What does this mean? It could mean that the organization needs to make a stronger effort to collect payment from its customers on a timely basis. Or it could mean that services were provided to patients who can't pay. The statement of cash flows highlights the fact that if receivables continue to grow at this rate, the organization will run out of cash, probably before the end of the next year. Although there is no crisis yet, there may be unless we take this situation into account in managing the organization and in planning for cash inflows and outflows for the coming year.

In the previous chapters we have followed the basic course of accounting events. Transactions get recorded via debit and credits in a journal using a chart of accounts. In turn, the journal entries get aggregated into the financial statements that we reviewed in this chapter. The next step in the accounting process is the audit of our financial statements by outside independent certified public accountants.

KEY CONCEPTS

Ledger—A book (or computer memory file) in which we keep track of the impact of financial events on each account. The ledger can provide us with the balance in any account at any point in time.

Operating statement preparation—The operating statement is directly prepared from the year-end ledger balances of the revenue and expense accounts.

Balance sheet preparation—Ledger account balances can be used to provide an analysis of changes in net asset accounts. This analysis, together with other ledger account balances, is used to prepare the balance sheet.

Statement of cash flows—This statement shows the sources and uses of the organization's cash. It specifically shows cash from operating, investing, and financing activities. It can be prepared under two alternative methods:

a. *the direct method*—Lists the change in cash caused by each account.

b. *the indirect method*—Starts with net income as an estimate of cash flow, and makes a series of adjustments to net income to determine cash flow from operating activities.

TEST YOUR KNOWLEDGE

See **www.jbpub.com/catalog/0763726753/supplements.htm.**

CHAPTER 8

The Role of the Outside Auditor

The stock market crash of 1929 brought to light substantial inadequacies in financial reporting. Investigations of bankrupt companies showed numerous arithmetic errors and cases of undetected fraud. These investigations also disclosed the common use of a widely varying set of accounting practices. A principal outcome of these investigations was that the newly formed Securities and Exchange Commission (SEC) required that publicly held companies annually issue a report to stockholders. The report must contain financial statements prepared by the organization's management and audited by a certified public accountant (CPA).

SEC rules are aimed at publicly-held for-profit companies (those with stockholders). Do not-for-profit health care organizations have to worry about having CPA-audited financial statements? Yes. Health care organizations are subject to a variety of rules and regulations that lead to the need for audited statements. For one thing, annual cost reports that must be provided to third-party payers often require that an audited set of financial statements be submitted as part of the report. If the health care organization issues bonds to raise funds for a capital project, the bondholders are entitled to audited statements. Banks often will not lend money without seeing audited statements. Even suppliers may require audited statements before selling to a health care provider on credit.

Annual reports are frequently referred to as *certified reports* or *certified statements,* although, in fact, it is the outside auditor who has been certified, not the statements themselves. Each state licenses CPAs and in granting the license certifies them as experts in accounting and auditing. The CPA gives an expert opinion regarding the financial statements of a company. There is no certification of correctness of the financial statements.

What exactly is the CPA's role in performing an audit? Well, some people consider the CPA to be the individual who walks out onto the field of battle after the fighting has died down and the smoke has cleared, and proceeds to shoot the wounded. CPAs have always been respected individuals, but in their role as auditors they tend to be seen in a rather unpleasant light, as the foregoing analogy indicates. This is largely because of a lack of understanding of what the CPA's role really is. The SEC, in requiring audited statements, was particularly concerned with arithmetic accuracy and the use of a clear, consistent set of accounting practices.

Ultimately, the SEC's desire is that a reliable set of financial statements, one that presents a "fair representation" of what has occurred, is given to the users of financial statement information. Those users include stockholders, bankers, suppliers, and other individuals. The CPA's focus is on the financial statements rather than on individual employees in the organization. Errors occur as long as humans are involved in the accounting process. The CPA has no interest in discrediting individuals. The CPA merely wants to ensure that the most significant of the errors are discovered and corrected.

THE AUDIT

The Management Letter and Internal Control

In performing an audit, the CPA checks for arithmetic accuracy. In performing this check, the external auditor focuses on the system rather than the individual.

Consider a system in which an individual is issuing invoices to insurance companies based on patients' medical records. The individual takes a copy of a medical record from the in box, records the dollar amounts and issues the invoice (or bill), and places the medical record in the out box to be brought back to the medical records department. Again and again, over and over, this same mechanical process is repeated. Occasionally the clerk takes the medical record, sips some coffee, and puts the document in the out box without having issued an invoice. Errors happen.

The auditor does not try to discover every such error; the cost of reexamining every financial transaction is prohibitive. Instead, by sampling some fraction of the documents processed, the auditor attempts to determine how often errors are occurring and how large they tend to be. The goal is to see if a material error exists.

What if the accountant feels that the clerk is making too many errors and the potential for a material misstatement may exist? The clerk must be fired and replaced with a more conscientious individual, right? No, wrong. Humans all make errors and the accountant wants the system to acknowledge that fact. The focus is on what accountants call the *internal control* of the accounting system. Basically, adequate internal control means that the system is designed in such a way as to catch and correct the majority of errors automatically, before the auditor arrives on the scene.

In our example with the clerk, the solution to the problem may be to have the clerk initial each document immediately after he or she processes the invoice. A second individual then reviews the documents to see that all have been initialed. Those that haven't been initialed are sent back for verification of whether an invoice was issued and for correction if need be. Errors can still occur—initialing the document after sipping the coffee, even though the invoice hasn't been processed—but they are less likely and should occur less frequently.

The auditor issues an internal control memo, often called a *management letter,* which points out the internal control weaknesses to management. Although there may be some expense involved for the organization to follow some of the recommendations, the inducement is that of reduced audit fees. Internal control weaknesses require an expanded audit so that the CPA can ascertain whether a material misstatement does exist. If the internal control is improved, the auditor feels more comfortable relying on the client's system and less audit testing is required. The management letter is given to the organization's top management and is not ordinarily disclosed to the public.

Fraud and Embezzlement

In an organization with good internal control, fraud and embezzlement are made difficult through a system of checks and balances. The auditor does not consider it to be a part of his or her job to detect all frauds. In fact, many cases of embezzlement are virtually impossible to uncover.

Although no statistics exist, it is likely that discovered embezzlements in this country amount to only the tip of the iceberg of what is really occurring. It is usually the greedy embezzlers that are caught. The modest embezzlers have an excellent chance of going undetected, especially if collusion among several employees exists.

A common misperception is that embezzlement leaves a hole in the bankbook. All of a sudden we go to withdraw money from our bank account and find that a million dollars is missing. This sort of open embezzlement is really the exception, not the rule.

Consider an individual whose job is to approve bills for payment. Suppose he was to print up stationary for Bill's Roofing Repair and send an invoice for $400 to his organization. What happens? He receives the invoice at work and approves it for payment. Large payments may require second approval. Therefore, larger embezzlements may require a partner if they are to go undetected.

Who is likely to question a small repair bill in a large organization? Or perhaps a series of small bills for office supplies? Our embezzler could be running 10 phony companies. One can easily conceive of an employee who, upon retirement after 40 years of apparently faithful service, admits to having charged the firm $1,000 a year for the last 35 years for maintenance and supply for a water cooler in the southern plant, even though the southern plant never had a water cooler.

Doesn't this type of embezzlement cause a cash shortage? No! We record the roofing repair expense or water cooler expense and reduce the cash account by the amount of the payment. Can the auditor issue his report on the financial statements of this company without discovering the fraud? Certainly. But then, doesn't that result in a material misstatement in the financial statements? Probably not, for several reasons.

First, the modest thief, not choosing to draw unwanted attention, is unlikely to steal a material amount of money. Second, the money is being correctly reported as an expense. We are calling the expense a roofing repair expense when, in fact, it should be called miscellaneous embezzlement expense. There would be no impact on the balance sheet nor on the organization's net income if we were to correct this misclassification! The cash account isn't overstated because the account was appropriately reduced when we paid the expense. The income isn't overstated because we did record an expense, even if we didn't correctly identify its cause.

How can the fraud be detected? If we send a letter to Bill's Roofing Repair and ask if their invoice was a bona fide bill, we will likely get an affirmative response, albeit coming from the embezzler himself. If we directly ask the employee if he approved the bill for payment, he will say yes, because he did approve it for payment to himself. To really see if this type of embezzlement is going on, we would have to trace each bill back to the individual in the organization who originally ordered the work done or the goods purchased. Unfortunately, the cost of the audit work involved is likely to far exceed the amount likely to have been embezzled.

The result is that the auditor tests some documents in an effort to scare the timid, but it is possible for numerous small frauds to go undetected. The auditor is also likely to suggest in the management letter that large payments require two approvals. This makes embezzlement of large amounts less likely unless there is collusion among at least two employees.

The Auditor's Report

In addition to the management letter, the auditor issues a letter to the Board of Directors or Trustees of the organization. This *opinion letter* generally has three standard paragraphs that are reproduced almost verbatim in most auditors' reports. Alternatively, some auditors combine the information from these three paragraphs into one longer paragraph. You might find it interesting to compare the auditor's letter from your organization's financial statement in the following sample letter.

Report of the Independent Auditors

To the Directors of Healthy Hospital:

We have audited the accompanying balance sheets of Healthy Hospital as of December 31, 2006 and 2007, and the related statements of operations, net assets, and cash flow for the years then ended. These financial statements are the responsibility of the Company's management. Our responsibility is to express an opinion on these financial statements based on our audits.

We conducted our audits in accordance with generally accepted auditing standards. Those standards require that we plan and perform the audit to obtain reasonable assurance about whether the financial statements are free of material misstatement. An audit includes examining, on a test basis, evidence supporting the amounts and disclosures in the financial statements. An audit also includes assessing the accounting principles used and significant estimates made by management, as well as evaluating the overall financial statement presentation. We believe that our audits provide a reasonable basis for our opinion.

In our opinion, the financial statements referred to above present fairly, in all material respects, the financial position of Healthy Hospital as of December 31, 2006 and 2007, and the results of its operations and its cash flows for the years then ended, in conformity with generally accepted accounting principles.

Finkler and Ward, CPAs
April 8, 2008

These three paragraphs are the standard *clean* opinion report. The first paragraph is referred to as the *opening* or *introductory* paragraph. The second paragraph is the *scope* paragraph. The third paragraph is the *opinion* paragraph. If there are any additional paragraphs, they are unusual and represent circumstances that require further explanation.

The opening paragraph serves to inform the users of the financial statements that an audit was performed. In some cases, auditors perform consulting or other services aside from audits. The opening paragraph also indicates explicitly that the organization's management bears the ultimate responsibility for the contents of the financial statements.

The scope paragraph describes the breadth or scope of work undertaken as a basis for forming an opinion on the financial statements. This paragraph explains the type of procedures auditors follow in carrying out an audit. Note that just as organizations must follow generally accepted accounting principles (GAAP) in preparing their statements, CPAs must follow generally accepted auditing standards in auditing those statements.

The opinion paragraph describes whether the financial statements provide a fair representation of the financial position, results of operations, and cash flows of the company, in the opinion of the auditor. A *clean* opinion, such as this one, indicates that in the opinion of the auditor, exercising due professional care, there is sufficient evidence of conformity to GAAP, and there is no condition requiring further clarification. This paragraph does not contend that the financial statements are completely correct. It does not even certify that there are no material misstatements. The CPA merely gives an expert opinion.

Note that the opinion of the CPA is that the financial statements are a fair representation of the organization's financial position. This is a somewhat audacious remark. Considering the intangible assets that often are not recorded on the financial statements despite their potentially significant value, and considering that plant, property, and equipment are recorded on the balance sheet at their cost, even though their value today may be far in excess of cost, you have to have a lot of nerve to say the statements are fair.

The key is that the accountant merely says the statements are a fair presentation in accordance with GAAP. In other words, this *fairness* is not meant to imply fair in any absolute meaning of the word *fair*.

Certainly this creates a problem in that many users of the financial statements are unfamiliar with the implications of GAAP. Such individuals may interpret the word *fair* in a broader sense than is intended. This is why it is vital that in looking at an annual report an individual read the notes to the financial statements as well as the statements themselves. Later in the book we discuss the notes to the financial statements in some detail.

The auditor may issue an *adverse, qualified,* or *disclaimer* opinion, if it is not possible to issue a clean opinion. An *adverse opinion* is a severe statement. It indicates that the auditor believes that the organization's financial statements are not presented fairly, in accordance with GAAP. A *qualified opinion* indicates that the financial statements are a fair representation in conformity with GAAP, except as relates to a specific particular area.

In some cases, the audit opinion letter also contains additional paragraphs containing explanations. This is generally the case if there is a significant uncertainty or a material change in the application of GAAP. Such paragraphs highlight special circumstances that might be of particular concern to the users of the financial statements. An example of a significant uncertainty is a lawsuit of such magnitude that, if the case is lost, it might cause the organization to become insolvent. Also, a material change in GAAP must be reported because it makes the current financial statement no longer completely comparable to the previous ones for the same company. The presence of more than the standard opening, scope, and opinion paragraphs should alert the user to exercise special care in interpreting the numbers reported in the financial statements.

The Management Report

It is common practice for the annual report of the organization to include not only the organization's financial statements and an auditor's report, but also a management report. In contrast to the management letter written by the CPA and given to the organization's management, the management report is written by the organization's management and is addressed to the readers of the annual report.

The management report explains that although the financial statements have been audited by an independent CPA, ultimately they are the responsibility of the organization's management. The report also discusses the organization's system of internal control and the role of its audit committee. The audit committee, consisting of members of the Board of Directors, has the responsibility for supervising the accounting, auditing, and other financial reporting matters of the organization.

Audit Failures

From time to time a major scandal hits the newspapers because an audit fails to provide users of financial statements with appropriate or timely information. The health industry financial community was finally recovering from the Allegheny Health System bankruptcy when the Health South scandal occurred. When events such as these happen, there are four principal issues to be considered: internal accounting systems, disclosure rules, auditor oversight, and ethics.

Internal Accounting Systems

One possible cause of situations such as the Allegheny bankruptcy is that the accounting systems at Allegheny were inadequate. Perhaps revenues that were not real were being inappropriately recorded and the accounting system was not designed well enough to pick it up.

Disclosure Rules

A second possible problem is that the existing rules for disclosure have loopholes that do not require all questionable practices to be disclosed. Usually after a highly visible event such as the Allegheny bankruptcy, the disclosure rules are reviewed, and the Financial Accounting Standards Board (FASB) and SEC make rule changes.

Auditor Oversight

CPAs are paid by the organization being audited. Desiring to keep earning their annual audit fees, auditors are sometimes convinced by their clients to allow questionable reporting practices. There is no doubt that the coming years will see changes in oversight of auditors to try to prevent future occurrences similar to Allegheny and Health South.

Ethics

Even with the best internal controls in place, at times auditors don't find everything, or worse yet, may even be complicit with management in perpetrating a fraud on their stockholders, lenders, employees, and the public. It is necessary to bear in mind that rules and accounting systems can't make up for a lack of ethical behavior on the part of the management or its outside auditor.

Avoiding Future Audit Failures

Clearly, to reduce the likelihood of such failures occurring again, several steps are needed. Auditors need to continue to work to help their clients improve their internal control systems. Regulators need to review and improve their disclosure rules. A better system of auditor oversight is essential. And finally, a culture of ethical behavior must be developed, or individuals will always find ways around the internal control systems and disclosure rules.

NEXT STEPS

Audited financial statements represent the completion of the financial accounting cycle. Transactions have been entered into journals. Journal entries have been aggregated into financial statements, and now those statements have been audited. So, what do all these financial statements really mean? The answer to this question lies in a thorough analysis of the financial statements. Unfortunately, before we are able to fully analyze the financial statements (see Chapter 13) we must first understand a few more critical accounting concepts. In Chapter 9 we introduce and explain depreciation and the effects this concept has on the financial statements. We then move to an explanation of inventory costing and how the value of inventory may directly affect the organization's bottom line.

KEY CONCEPTS

Audited financial statements—Presentation of the organization's financial position and its results of operations, in accordance with GAAP.

Management letter—Report to top management that makes suggestions for the improvement of internal control to reduce the likelihood of errors and undetected frauds or embezzlements.

Auditor's report—Letter from the outside auditor giving an opinion on whether or not the organization's financial statements are a fair presentation of the organization's results of operations, cash flows, and financial position in accordance with GAAP.

Management report—Letter from the organization's management that is part of the annual report.

TEST YOUR KNOWLEDGE

See www.jbpub.com/catalog/0763726753/supplements.htm.

CHAPTER 9

Depreciation: Having Your Cake and Eating It Too!

The *matching principle* of accounting requires that organizations use depreciation. Suppose we buy a machine with a 10-year useful life. This machine helps to produce services over its entire 10-year lifetime. Therefore, it generates revenues in each of those 10 years. The matching principle holds that we would be distorting the results of operations in all 10 years if we considered the entire cost of the machine to be an expense in the year in which it was acquired. We would be understating income in the first year and overstating it in subsequent years.

Instead of expensing the equipment, we consider it to be a long-term asset when it is acquired. As time passes and the equipment becomes used up, we allocate a portion of the original cost as an expense in each year. Thus, the revenue received each year related to the services provided by the machine is matched with some of the machine's cost.

Okay, if we have to do it that way, there is some intuitive rationale. But where is the financial decision? It seems as if there is little choice left for the financial manager. In fact, that is not true. There are several complicating factors. We must determine both the valuation to be used as a basis for each year's depreciation as well as the depreciation method. Although this sounds simple enough, it really involves a number of steps; we must ensure that all costs associated with the asset are captured, we must estimate both the expected life of the asset and what the asset will be worth at the end of its useful life (the *salvage value*), and finally we must determine whether the asset gets used up proportionally during its life. For-profit health care organizations must also ask what the tax implications are of the depreciation methods they decide to use. These issues make up the topic of this chapter. Figure 9-1 lays out the depreciation process that organizations go through to calculate depreciation. The components of the process are discussed below.

AMORTIZATION

Amortization is the spreading out of a cost over a period of time. It is a generic term used for any type of item that is being prorated over time. *Depreciation* is a specialized subset of amortization. Depreciation refers to the wearing out of a tangible asset such as a building or piece of equipment.

Some items don't wear out per se, and we don't refer to them as depreciating over time. For example, natural resources such as oil, gas, and coal are said to deplete. *Deplete* means to empty out, and this is essentially

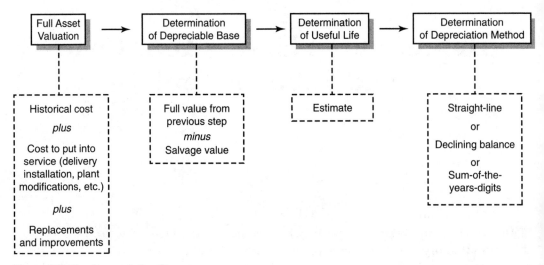

Figure 9-1 The Depreciation Process

what happens to a coal mine or oil well. Finally, some items neither deplete nor depreciate. For example, a patent loses its value over time. It doesn't break down, wear out, or empty out—it simply expires with the passage of time. When neither of the terms *depreciation* nor *depletion* is applicable, we refer to the item as *amortizing*. Therefore, for a patent, the annual reduction in value is referred to as *amortization expense*. This chapter speaks exclusively of depreciation, even though the principles generally apply in a similar fashion for assets to be depleted or amortized.

ASSET VALUATION FOR DEPRECIATION

The first step in the depreciation process is the determination of the full cost of the asset to be depreciated. As you may remember from Chapter 5, accountants have a habit of being able to look at a particular asset and come up with a number of different values for it. The process of determining "the" value that will be used in financial statements is referred to as *valuation*. In the

case of depreciation, valuation of the asset being depreciated is critical. This first step in the depreciation process sets the stage for all the calculations that follow.

Asset valuation for depreciation basically follows the rules of historical cost. Chapter 5 stated that the historical or acquisition cost of an asset is simply what we paid for the item when we acquired it. However, for depreciation purposes, determination of asset cost is somewhat more complex.

The first problem that arises is the issue of what to do with the costs of putting an asset into productive service. For example, suppose that we purchase a machine for $40,000, and we cannot use the machine without modifying our electrical system. If we pay an electrician $2,000 to run a heavy-duty power line to the spot where the machine will be located, is that a current period expense? No; according to generally accepted accounting principles (GAAP), the cost of the electrical work provides us with benefits over the entire useful life of the machine. Therefore, matching requires that we spread the cost of the electrical work over the same period as the life of the machine. The way that is handled is by adding the cost of the electrical work to the cost of the equipment. Instead of our equipment showing a cost of $40,000, it has a cost of $42,000 and we depreciate that amount over its lifetime.

In fact, all costs to put an item into service are added to the cost of that item so that they can be matched with the revenues over the useful life of the asset. This includes freight on the purchase, insurance while in transit to our facility, new fixtures, and plant modifications. Further, although repairs and maintenance are current period expenses, replacements and improvements to an asset must be added to the cost and depreciated over the life remaining at the time of the replacement or improvement. Replacements and improvements are simply expenditures that extend the useful life of the asset, improve its speed or quality, or reduce its operating costs.

If a motor burns out, is its replacement a routine repair expense charged to the current year, or is the cost of the replacement *capitalized* (that is, added to the cost of a long-term item shown on the balance sheet)? That depends on the circumstances. Do motors burn out quite regularly, or is it a rare event? Regular replacement may well be a repair, but infrequent major overhauls are capitalized. However, there is no clear right or wrong answer in many instances.

As you can see, determining the full cost of the asset to be depreciated is not as simple as identifying what was paid directly for the particular asset. Ultimately, the cost of the asset listed on the balance sheet (and thereby depreciated over its life) is a combination of the direct acquisition cost of the asset, all indirect costs associated with getting the asset into service, and all subsequent replacements and improvements.

Equipment tends to have acquisition and installation costs, whereas property and physical plant items tend to have acquisition and improvement costs. A roof is another common example of a capital improvement. Ongoing roof maintenance (replacing a shingle or two) is a current operating expense. Replacing the entire roof is an improvement that extends the use of the asset and therefore needs to be added to the value of that asset and subsequently depreciated. Determining the full value of an asset is not only critical to the calculation of depreciation, it is more complicated than most people think.

The Depreciable Base

Our problems are not yet over. How much of the asset's cost do we depreciate? Your first reaction may well be to say the entire cost, including the various additions to the purchase price that we have just discussed. This is basically true, except that there is still a matching problem. We wish to depreciate property that wears out over the course of its use to get a portion of its cost to assign to each period in which the asset helps generate revenues. However, we only want to match against revenues those resources that actually get used up. We don't necessarily consume 100% of most assets.

Suppose we bought a machine with a 10-year expected life at a cost of $40,000, including all of the costs to put it into service. Suppose further that after 10 years we expect to be able to sell the machine for $4,000. Then we really have not used up $40,000 of resources over the 10 years. We have used up only $36,000 and we still have a $4,000 asset left over. This $4,000 value is referred to as the machine's *salvage value.* Therefore, from an accounting perspective, we depreciate a machine by an amount equal to its cost less its anticipated salvage value. That difference is referred to as its *depreciable base*.

The salvage value has to be estimated—at best, it is an educated guess. Your accountant reviews the reasonableness of your salvage value estimates for financial statement preparation.

Asset Life

The next step in the depreciation process is to determine how long an asset lasts. We attempt to depreciate an asset over its useful life. If we depreciate it over a period longer or shorter than its useful life, we don't obtain an accurate matching between revenues and the expenses incurred to generate those revenues. However, we can only guess an asset's true useful life. Often we see equipment that lasts well after the estimated useful life. This is not surprising, considering the GAAP of conservatism. Better to write off an asset too quickly and understate its true value than to write it off too slowly (anticipating a longer life than ultimately results) and overstate its value.

What happens if we are still using the asset after its estimated useful life is over? We stop taking further depreciation. The role of depreciation is to allocate some of the cost of the asset into each of a number of years or accounting periods. Once we have allocated all of the cost (less the salvage value), we simply continue to use the asset with no further depreciation. That means we have revenues without depreciation expense matched against them. That is simply a result of a matching based on estimates rather than being based on perfect foreknowledge.

What if we sell the asset for more than its salvage value? That presents no problem—we can record a gain for the difference between the selling price and the asset's *book value*. The book value of an asset is the amount paid for it, less the amount of depreciation already taken. Thus, if we bought our machine for $40,000, and sold it after 10 years during which we had taken $36,000 of depreciation, its book value is $4,000. According to our financial records, or books, its value is $4,000. If we sell it for $10,000, there is a gain of $6,000.

What if the asset becomes obsolete after 3 years owing to technological change and it is sold at that time for $1,000? Assuming we were depreciating it at a rate of $3,600 a year (to arrive at $36,000 of depreciation over 10 years), then we would have taken $10,800 of depreciation (3 years at $3,600 per year) during those first 3 years. The book value ($40,000 cost less $10,800 of accumulated depreciation) is $29,200, and at a sale price of $1,000, we record a loss of $28,200.

Accumulated Depreciation

In Chapter 7, the balance sheet had a line for *Plant and Equipment, Net*. This means the cost of the plant and equipment, less any depreciation that has been charged to that plant and equipment while we have owned it. The full amount of depreciation that has been taken on a piece of depreciable property over all the years you have owned it is called *accumulated depreciation*. It is important to distinguish between each year's depreciation expense and the accumulated depreciation.

Take the equipment discussed above. The acquisition cost was $40,000, it has a $4,000 salvage value, and therefore a $36,000 depreciable base. Assuming the 10-year useful life, for the next 10 years the operating statement will show a $3,600 depreciation expense each year.

How does the equipment appear on the balance sheet? At the end of the first year, it appears as $36,400, net. This is the $40,000 cost, less the first year's depreciation expense. By the end of the second year, we have taken a total of $7,200 of depreciation expense (i.e., $3,600 per year for 2 years). That $7,200 is referred to as the accumulated depreciation for that piece of equipment. The net value of the equipment is now shown on the balance sheet as $32,800 (i.e., the $40,000 cost, less the $7,200 of accumulated depreciation).

STRAIGHT-LINE VERSUS ACCELERATED DEPRECIATION

The final step in the depreciation process is the determination of the depreciation method that is used to calculate the annual depreciation expense. In the previous example we noted that $7,200 of depreciation had been taken over 2 years, if we assume depreciation of $3,600 per year. The $3,600 figure is based on *straight-line* depreciation. It assumes that we take an equal share of the total depreciation each year during the asset's life.

In fact, we have choices for how we calculate the depreciation. The straight-line approach is just one of several methods available. Not all equipment declines in productive value equally in each year of its useful life. Consider a machine that has a capacity of 1 million units of output over its lifetime. If it is run three shifts a day, it will be used up substantially quicker than if it is run only one shift a day. The *units of production* or *units of activity* method of depreciation bases each year's depreciation on the proportion of the machine's total productive capacity that has been used in that year. For instance, if the machine produces 130,000 units in a year, and its estimated total lifetime capacity is 1 million, we take 13% (130,000 divided by 1,000,000) of the cost less salvage value as the depreciation for that year. Of course, this method entails substantial extra bookkeeping to keep track of annual production.

Two other methods exist that are commonly used—the *declining balance method* (really this is a group of similar methods as discussed below) and the *sum-of-the-years' digits* method. These are called *accelerated* methods. The basic philosophy behind these methods is that some assets are likely to decline in value more rapidly in the early years of their life than in the later years. A car is an excellent example. If we consider the decline in value for a car, it is largest in its first year, not quite as large in the following year, and eventually tails off to a point where there is relatively little decline per year in the latter part of its life.

COMPARISON OF THE DEPRECIATION METHODS

We use an example to demonstrate the principal depreciation methods and to allow us to compare the results using each method. Assume that we buy a machine for $40,000 and we have $8,000 of costs to put the machine into service. We expect the machine to have a useful life of 6 years and a salvage value of $6,000.

The straight-line (SL) method first calculates the depreciable base, which is the cost less salvage. In this case, the cost is the $40,000 price plus the $8,000 to put the machine into service. The salvage value is $6,000, so the depreciable base is $42,000 ($40,000 + $8,000 − $6,000). The base is then allocated equally among the years of the asset's life. For a 6-year life, the depreciation is 1/6 of the $42,000 each year, or $7,000 per year. The straight-line method is rather straightforward.

The declining balance method accelerates the amount of depreciation taken in the early years and reduces the amount taken in the later years. When someone refers to accelerated depreciation, he or she is not referring to a shortening of the asset life for depreciation purposes. The life remains 6 years under the accelerated methods. Declining balance represents a group of methods. We start with double declining balance (DDB), also referred to as 200% declining balance. We discuss the other declining balance methods below.

The DDB approach starts out with a depreciable base equal to the asset cost ignoring salvage value. The cost is multiplied, not by 1/6 as in the SL method, but by a rate that is double the SL rate. In this case we multiply the depreciable base by 2 times 1/6, or by 2/6. Hence the word *double* in the name of this method. If we take 2/6 of $48,000 (remember that cost includes the various costs to get the machine into service, and that this method ignores salvage value), we get $16,000 of depreciation for the first year. At that rate, the asset will be fully depreciated in just 3 years, and we've said that accelerated methods generally do not shorten the asset life!

Therefore, we need some device to prevent the depreciation from remaining at that high level of $16,000 per year. This device is the *declining balance*. Each year we subtract the previous year's depreciation from the existing depreciable base to get a new depreciable base. In this example, we start with a base of $48,000 and take $16,000 of depreciation in the first year. This means that in the second year there is a new depreciable base of $32,000 ($48,000 − $16,000). In the second year, our depreciation is 2/6 of $32,000, or $10,667. For year 3, we determine a new base equal to $32,000 less the depreciation of $10,667 in year 2. Thus, we have a new base of $21,334, and so on.

However, there is one caveat to this process. We cannot take more depreciation during the asset's life than the asset's cost

less its salvage value. In this problem, we can take no more than $42,000 of depreciation, regardless of the method chosen. We have achieved our goal of having higher depreciation in the early years and less in each succeeding year. The method, which doubles the SL rate, does have some intuitive appeal as an approach for getting the desired accelerated effect.

The declining balance family also includes 150% declining balance and 175% declining balance. In each of these methods, the only difference from the 200%, or DDB, is that the SL rate is multiplied by 150% or 175% instead of 200% to find the annual rate.

Sum-of-the-years' digits (SYD) is a similar accelerated method. SYD takes the cost less salvage, that is, $42,000, the same as SL, and multiplies it by a fraction that consists of the life of the asset divided by the sum of the digits in the years of the life of the asset. That sum consists of adding from one to the last year of the asset's life, inclusive. In our example, we add $1 + 2 + 3 + 4 + 5 + 6$, because the asset has a 6-year life. The sum of these digits is 21. Therefore, we multiply $42,000 by 6/21 (the life of the asset divided by the sum). This gives us first-year depreciation of $12,000.

In each succeeding year, we lower the numerator of the fraction by 1. That is, for year 2, the fraction becomes 5/21 and the depreciation amount is $10,000 ($42,000 × 5/21). For year 3, the fraction becomes 4/21 and the depreciation $8,000, and so on. It is hard to find any intuitive appeal to this manipulation. All we can say is that it does achieve the desired result of greater depreciation in the early years, and it does account for the proper amount of total depreciation.

Table 9-1 compares the three methods for this piece of equipment for its entire 6-year life. It is especially important to note that all three methods produce exactly the same total depreciation over the life of the asset.

Year	Straight-Line (SL)	Double Declining Balance (DDB)	Sum-of the-Years' Digits (SYD)
1	$ 7,000	$ 16,000	$ 12,000
2	7,000	10,667	10,000
3	7,000	7,111	8,000
4	7,000	4,741	6,000
5	7,000	3,160	4,000
6	7,000	321	2,000
Total	$ 42,000	$ 42,000	$ 42,000

Table 9-1 Comparison of Depreciation Methods

Ideally, in choosing a depreciation method for your organization, you select from among SL, declining balance, and SYD based on the method that most closely approximates the manner in which your particular resources are used up and become less productive. You need not use the same method for all of your depreciable property.

Many organizations simply choose the SL approach for reporting depreciation on their financial statements. The apparent reason for this is that it tends to cause net income to be higher in the early years than it would be using the accelerated methods and their high charges to depreciation expense.

Excel Template

Template 6 may be used to calculate straight-line and accelerated depreciation using your organization's data. The template is on the Web at www.jbpub.com.

For not-for-profit health care organizations, the depreciation process is now complete. The last step of the process, considering the implications of depreciation on taxes, is only applicable to the for-profit health care organizations. It is to the special tax treatment of depreciation that we now turn our attention.

MODIFIED ACCELERATED COST RECOVERY SYSTEM

The first and most important point that the reader should be aware of is that this is one place where you can actually have your cake and eat it too! For-profit health care organizations are not required to use the same methods of depreciation for reporting to the Internal Revenue Service (IRS) as they use for reporting to their stockholders. The implications of that are enormous. We can use straight-line depreciation on our financial statements, thus keeping our depreciation expense relatively low, and be able to tell our stockholders that we had a very fine year. Then we can use the IRS accelerated depreciation system, called the *modified accelerated cost recovery system* (MACRS), which accelerates depreciation, lowering income and taxes in the early years of an asset's life.

We highlight many of the important issues here. However, we can't stress strongly enough the benefits of consulting a tax expert. Tax law is an area that requires up-to-date expertise. The tax law changes constantly, not only because of congressional action, but also as a result of IRS rulings and interpretations and the results of court cases. No tax decisions should be made based solely on the information contained in this book.

The most important aspect of the IRS depreciation system is that it assigns shorter lives to assets. Generally these shorter lives are not used in preparation of financial statements for reports to stockholders. The law does give some leeway in extending the life of the asset by choosing a less accelerated approach, but most organizations find that the basic MACRS approach provides the quickest allowable deductions and lowest current tax payments, and is therefore beneficial in most cases. By accelerating a deduction, a profitable organization can push its tax payments off to the future, thus effectively getting an interest-free loan from the government.

Under MACRS, asset lives are substantially shorter than their useful life estimates, and salvage value is ignored until we actually dispose of the asset. The government-imposed lifetimes for depreciation under MACRS for different types of assets are 3, 5, 7, 10, 15, 20, 27.5, and 39 years.

The 3-, 5-, 7-, and 10-year classes are depreciated under the 200% or DDB system that substantially accelerates depreciation. The 15- and 20-year classes are depreciated using a 150% declining balance method. The 27.5- and 39-year classes are depreciated on a SL basis.

The MACRS 3-year category includes items such as tractors, some machine tools, and racehorses over 12 years old. Leave it to Congress!

The MACRS 5-year category includes property with a useful life of more than 4 but less than 10 years. This class specifically includes computers, cars, trucks, and research and experimental equipment.

The MACRS 7-year class includes property that has a life of 10 to 15 years. This generally includes office furniture and fixtures and property that does not explicitly fall into another category.

The MACRS 10-year class is for property with a life of 16 to 19 years. Included are vessels, barges, and tugs.

The MACRS 15-year class includes property with a life of 20 to 24 years. This category includes billboards, service station buildings, and land improvements.

The MACRS 20-year class is for property with a useful life of 25 years or more, such as utilities and sewers.

Residential rental property falls into the 27.5-year class, and most nonresidential real property has a class period of 39 years.

Although all of this may make your head swim, the government has kindly provided tables giving the percentage of the asset's cost to be taken as depreciation for tax purposes in each year of the asset's life. For example, Table 9-2 provides a table showing the portion of the asset to be depreciated each year under MACRS, for the 3- through 20-year classes. Note that the table contains 21 years because it is generally assumed that each asset (except real property) is put into service halfway into the year. The first and last years each contain only a half-year of depreciation. (It should be noted as an aside that there is a less favorable mid-quarter convention that applies if substantial portions of a year's assets are placed into service in the last 3 months of the tax year.)

Excel Template

Template 7 may be used to calculate MACRS depreciation for your organization. The template is included on the web at www.jbpub.com.

Tax law is complex and changes frequently. Do not file tax returns based on information from the use of this template without first consulting a tax expert.

In some instances, it is possible to deduct in 1 tax year approximately $100,000 of assets, rather than depreciating them under MACRS. This is an option available to the taxpayer for some types of property used in a trade or business. It is referred to as a *Section 179 expense.* The available deduction is phased out if more than approximately $400,000 worth of qualified property is placed into service during the tax year. To the extent that you can avail yourself of this rule, it can provide an even faster tax write-off of the asset than MACRS would generate.

Another tax issue concerns "Section 197 Intangibles." This refers to goodwill and other purchased intangibles. Firms may deduct the

Table 9-2 MACRS Schedule for Property Placed in Service after 1986

Year	3-Year Class	5-Year Class	7-Year Class	10-Year Class	15-Year Class	20-Year Class
1	33.33	20.00	14.29	10.00	5.00	3.750
2	44.45	32.00	24.49	18.00	9.50	7.219
3	14.81	19.20	17.49	14.40	8.55	6.677
4	7.41	11.52	12.49	11.52	7.70	6.177
5		11.52	8.93	9.22	6.93	5.713
6		5.76	8.92	7.37	6.23	5.285
7			8.93	6.55	5.90	4.888
8			4.46	6.55	5.90	4.522
9				6.56	5.91	4.462
10				6.55	5.90	4.461
11				3.28	5.91	4.462
12					5.90	4.461
13					5.91	4.462
14					5.90	4.461
15					5.91	4.462
16					2.95	4.461
17						4.462
18						4.461
19						4.462
20						4.461
21						2.231

cost of such intangibles as an expense for tax purposes on a SL basis over a 15-year period.

What's the bottom line to all this? Essentially, you can base the income you report to your stockholders on SL depreciation extended over the asset's useful life and using a salvage value, and at the same time, use the MACRS method for reporting to the IRS. Thus, you show your stockholders a net income that is higher than you show the IRS. You therefore report relatively high income to the owners (your bosses), and yet pay relatively low taxes because of the higher depreciation reported to the government. Have you actually reduced your tax payments, or just shifted them off to the future? That is a very interesting question and one that is the basis for the discussion of deferred taxes.

DEPRECIATION AND DEFERRED TAXES: ACCOUNTING MAGIC

We discussed the use of straight-line depreciation for financial statements and MACRS for the tax return. The fact that we can tell different depreciation stories to our stockholders and the IRS has interesting ramifications for the organization and its financial statements. It creates something called a *temporary difference.* Our financial records record taxes in a different year than our tax return does. This applies only to for-profit organizations because not-for-profit organizations are not subject to income taxes.

If we tell our stockholders that we had a good year, then they expect the organization to pay a lot of taxes on the profits we are currently making. Even if we don't pay those taxes now, but instead defer payment to the future, the matching principle seems to require that we record the tax expense based on our depreciation in our financial records, rather than when the IRS calculates the depreciation and taxes. In fact, that is exactly the case. Taxes are recorded on the organization's financial statements as tax expense and a liability, called a *deferred tax liability*. However, the implications of this deferred tax are quite unusual—almost magical.

Generally, if we can postpone payment of taxes, with no other change in the operation of our business in any respect, we should do so. For any one asset, the deferred tax liability represents an interest-free loan that is eventually repaid to the government. However, what is true for one asset is not necessarily true for the entire organization. For many companies, balances in the deferred tax account do not become zero, but rather grow continuously into the future.

This rather amazing result is simply explained. If we had one depreciable asset, over its lifetime we would first defer some tax and later repay it. But if we are constantly replacing equipment—buying new equipment as old equipment wears out—the deferral increase on the new assets offsets the deferral reduction on the old assets, often causing the deferral to effectively become a permanent interest-free loan. However, the magic of deferred taxes is not yet fully apparent.

Consider what happens for an organization that is growing. Such an organization is not only offsetting higher taxes on older equipment with deferred taxes on an equal amount of new equipment. The expansion in fixed assets causes the deferred liability to grow each year. For growing companies, the startling result is that deferred taxes represent both a growing and permanent interest-free loan. A bit of accounting magic.

KEY CONCEPTS

Matching—Depreciation is an attempt to match the cost of resources used up over a period longer than 1 year with the revenues those resources generate over their useful lifetime.

Amortization—Generic term for the spreading out of costs over a period of time. Depreciation is a special case of amortization.

Amounts to be depreciated—Cost of an asset, less its salvage value, is depreciated over the asset's useful life. The cost is the fair market value at the time of acquisition, plus costs to put the asset into service, plus the costs of improvements made to the asset.

Depreciate methods—Asset may be depreciated on a SL basis, resulting in an equal amount of depreciation each year, or by an accelerated method, which results in greater depreciation in the earlier years of the asset's life. Two common accelerated depreciation methods are DDB and SYD.

Modified Accelerated Cost Recovery System (MACRS)—Depreciation method used for tax reporting.

Deferred taxes—If the pretax income reported to stockholders is more than that reported to the IRS, then a tax deferral will arise; that is, some of our current tax expense becomes a liability to be paid at some unstated time in the future, rather than being paid currently.

TEST YOUR KNOWLEDGE

See www.jbpub.com/catalog/0763726753/supplements.htm.

CHAPTER 10

Inventory Costing: The Accountant's World of Make-Believe

THE INVENTORY EQUATION

Inventories are a stock of goods held for use in production, delivery of services, or for sale. Retailers and wholesalers, like drugstores and medical supply stores, have merchandise inventory. They buy a product basically in the same form as that in which it is sold. Manufacturers, like pharmaceutical companies or medical device makers, have several classes of inventory—raw materials that are used in the manufacturing process to make a final product; work in process that consists of goods on which production has begun but has not yet been finished; and finished goods that are complete and awaiting sale.

Just as there is a basic equation of accounting, there is a basic equation for keeping track of inventory and its cost:

Beginning   Units   Units   Ending
Inventory + Purchased − Sold = Inventory
(BI)   (P)   (S)   (EI)

This equation can be understood from a reasonably intuitive point of view. Consider an organization selling syringes. At the start of the year, it has 2,000 syringes. During the year, it buys 8,000 syringes. If it sells 6,000 syringes, how many are left at the end of the year?

BI	+	P	−	S	=	EI
2,000	+	8,000	−	6,000	=	4,000

We can readily see that there should be 4,000 syringes on hand at year end.

PERIODIC VERSUS PERPETUAL INVENTORY METHODS

Organizations must make a major decision about the way in which they intend to keep track of the four items in the inventory equation. This year's beginning inventory is always last year's ending inventory. All accounting systems are designed so as to keep track of purchases. A problem centers on the cost of goods sold and ending inventory. (Because many health care organizations *use* inventory in the delivery of services, we sometimes refer to the traditional *cost of goods sold* as *cost of goods used*.)

If we wish, we can keep track of specifically how many and which items in our inventory are used. However, this requires a fair amount of bookkeeping. And in the end, it may not be worth the cost. Consider a community clinic that stocks hundreds (or thousands) of aspirin. Maintaining a running count of how many aspirin are distributed may require paying a clerk just to watch and count the aspirin.

A far simpler approach is to simply wait until year end and then count what is left. Once we know the ending inventory, we can use our inventory equation to determine how many aspirin were distributed. For example, if we started with 2,000 aspirin and purchased 8,000, then a year-end count of 4,000 on hand indicates that we distributed 6,000 during the year.

$$BI \quad + \quad P \quad - \quad S \quad = \quad EI$$

If:

$$2,000 \quad + \quad 8,000 \quad - \quad S \quad = \quad 4,000$$

then

$$S \quad = \quad 6,000$$

This method is called the *periodic method of inventory*. It requires us to take a physical count to find out what we have on hand at any point in time. It gets this name because we keep track of inventory from time to time, or periodically.

A major weakness of the periodic system is that, at any point in time, we don't know how much inventory we've used and how much we have left. Therefore, our control over our inventory is rather limited. If running out of an item creates a serious problem, this method is inadequate.

There are several easy solutions to that problem in some situations. If, for example, the aspirin are kept in a bin, we can paint a stripe two thirds of the way down the bin. When we see the stripe, we know it's time to reorder. Bookstores often solve this problem by placing a reorder card in a book near the bottom of the pile. When that book is sold an order is made to replenish the stock.

The periodic method has other weaknesses as well. Although we calculate a figure for units used based on the three other elements of the inventory equation, we don't know for sure that just because a unit of inventory isn't on hand, it was used. It may have broken, spoiled, expired, or been stolen.

An alternative to periodic inventory accounting is the *perpetual method* for keeping track of units of inventory. Just as the name implies, you always, or perpetually, know how much inventory you have, because you specifically record each item. This method is appropriate for companies selling relatively few high-priced items. In such cases, it is relatively inexpensive to keep track of each sale relative to the dollar value of the sale. Furthermore, control of inventory tends to be a more important issue with high-priced items.

Which of the two methods is considered more useful? Clearly the perpetual method gives more information and better control. However, it also adds substantially to bookkeeping costs. Most firms would choose perpetual if they could get it for the same money as periodic, but typically they can't. The result is a management decision as to whether the extra benefits of perpetual are worth the extra cost.

Computers have made significant inroads in allowing organizations to switch to perpetual inventory without incurring prohibitively high costs. For example, supermarkets were a classic example of the type of organization that couldn't afford perpetual inventory. Imagine a checkout clerk in the supermarket manually writing down each item as it's sold. The clerk rings up one can of peas, and then turns and writes down "one 6-ounce can of Green Midget peas." Then the clerk rings up one can of corn, and turns and writes down, "one 4-ounce can of House Brand corn," and so on. At the end of the day, another clerk would tally up the manual logs of each checkout clerk. The cost of this would be enormous. In such a situation, an organization would just keep track of total dollars of sales, and would take periodic inventories to see what is still on hand. Yet supermarkets run on extremely tight margins, so they can ill afford to run out of goods, nor can they afford the carrying cost of excess inventory.

Supermarkets were among the leaders in adopting use of bar codes. These computer-sensitive markings allow the store to save the cost of stamping the price on goods. The computer that reads the bar code knows how much the price of each item is, so the clerk no longer needs to see a stamped price. It also allows the clerk to ring up the goods at a much faster pace. Finally, it automatically updates the inventory. In many supermarkets using this system, the cash register tape gives you more information than just the price. Not only does it tell you that you bought a 4-ounce container of yogurt, but also that it was blueberry yogurt. That detailed information tells the supermarket's main computer the size, brand, and flavor of yogurt to be restocked. The potential time saved in stamping prices on goods and in the checkout process can offset much of the cost of the computer system.

Many larger health care organizations, especially hospitals, have adopted bar coding and perpetual inventory systems. In health care, the use of bar codes has moved beyond the tracking of inventory to the tracking of medical records, services provided, and even the tracking of patients as they move throughout the hospital.

It should be noted that even on a perpetual system there is a need to physically count inventory from time to time (typically at least once a year). The perpetual method keeps track of what was used. If there is a pilferage or breakage, our inventory records will not be correct. However, when we use a perpetual system, we know what we should have. When we count our inventory, we can determine the extent to which goods that have not been used are missing.

THE PROBLEM OF INFLATION

The periodic and perpetual methods of inventory tracking help us to determine the quantity of goods on hand and the quantity used. We must also determine which units were used and which units are on hand. Consider the following situation:

	Quantity	Cost ($)
Beginning Inventory	20,000	200 each
Purchase March 1	20,000	220 each
Purchase June 1	20,000	240 each
Purchase September 1	20,000	260 each
Use during Year	60,000	

How many units are left in stock? Clearly from our basic inventory equation the answer to that is 20,000. Beginning inventory of 20,000 units, plus the purchases of 60,000 units, less the use of 60,000 units leaves ending inventory of 20,000 units. What is the value of those 20,000 units? Here a problem arises. Which 20,000 units are left? Does it matter? From an accounting point of view it definitely does matter. In Chapter 3, we noted that generally accepted accounting principles require us to value items on the balance sheet at their cost. To know the cost of our remaining units, we must know which units we used and which are still on hand. This requires the manager to make some assumptions, referred to as *cost-flow assumptions.*

This is particularly important during periods of high inflation. Recently, inflation has been modest, but at some point in the near future the rate of inflation may accelerate. Therefore managers need an understanding of the impact of the cost-flow assumptions that they make.

COST-FLOW ASSUMPTIONS

The methods for determining which units were used and which are on hand are referred to as cost-flow assumptions. There are four major alternative cost-flow assumptions.

Specific Identification

This is the accountant's ideal. It entails physically tagging each unit in some way so that we can specifically identify the units on hand with their cost. Then, when a periodic inventory is taken, we can determine the cost of all the units on hand and therefore deduce the cost of the units used.

As you might expect, for most organizations such tagging would create a substantial additional bookkeeping cost. Think of the community clinic not just trying to keep track of how many aspirin are used, but also the specific aspirin. Can any type of business go to this effort? Certainly some can—typically those organizations that keep close track of serial numbers for the items used.

For example, a drug store must keep track of specific lot numbers for each medication in stock. By doing so, they can keep track of specifically which pills from which lot were dispensed and which specific pills remain in inventory. Similarly, hospitals must track which specific medical device (such as a pacemaker) is implanted into each patient in case there is a recall of that device.

First-In, First-Out

The second cost-flow approach is called *first-in, first-out*, and is almost always referred to by the shorthand acronym FIFO. This method allows you to keep track of the flow of inventory without tagging each item. It is based on the fact that, in most industries, inventory moves in an orderly fashion. We can think of

a hospital that has medical supplies with an expiration date. Imagine that hospital as a building with a front door and a back door. New deliveries of merchandise are received at the back door and put on a conveyor belt. They move along the conveyor belt and right out the front door. We would never have occasion to skip 1 unit ahead of the other items already on the conveyor belt ahead of it.

A good example of FIFO is a dairy. It is clear that the dairy would always prefer to sell the milk that comes out of the cow today, before they sell the milk that the cow produces tomorrow. We've all seen in the supermarket that the freshest milk is put on the back of the shelf. Of course, we know the fresh milk is in the back so we sometimes reach back to get it. But then, they know we know so they sometimes.... Nevertheless, the point is clear—the supermarket's desire is for us to buy the oldest milk first; they want to sell the milk in a FIFO fashion.

In health care, the closest example to the dairy is a drug store that stocks refrigerated medication that has expiration dates. Clearly, like the milk, the goal is to dispense the oldest medication first. The first medication placed in the refrigerator needs to be the first out.

In most industries there is a desire to avoid winding up with old, shopworn, obsolete, dirty goods. Therefore, FIFO makes reasonable sense as an approach for processing inventory.

Weighted Average

The weighted average (WA) approach to inventory cost flows assumes that our entire inventory is commingled and there is no way to determine which units were used. For example, consider the community clinic and the aspirin again. Suppose the clinic purchases their first batch of aspirin for $.10 per pill and all the pills are dumped in a large bin. A week later, when the bin is half full, they reordered the aspirin, but this time the batch cost $.14 per pill and again, the pills are dumped into the bin. We now dispense two pills to a patient; are we dispensing pills that cost $.10 or $.14? Because there is really no way to know, the WA method assumes that all of the pills have been thoroughly mixed, and therefore the pills being dispensed cost $.12 per pill. This method is appropriate whenever inventory gets stirred or mixed together and it is physically impossible to determine what has been used.

Last-In, First-Out

The last of the four methods of cost flow for inventory is last-in, first-out (LIFO), which has received much attention in the last decade. The LIFO method is just the reverse of the FIFO method. It assumes that the last goods we receive are the first goods we use. In the case of the dairy it would mean that we always would try to sell the freshest milk first and keep the older, souring milk in our warehouse.

Does the LIFO method make sense for any industries at all? Yes. In fact it is the logical approach to use for any industry that piles their goods up as they arrive, and then uses from the top of the pile. For example, a company mining coal or making chemicals frequently piles them up and them simply sells from the top of the pile. However, for most organizations it doesn't provide a very logical inventory movement. Nevertheless, a large number of organizations have shifted from the FIFO method to the LIFO method. Why?

Comparisons of the LIFO and FIFO Cost-Flow Assumptions

Financial statements are not ideally suited for inflationary environments. During infla-

tion, we have problems trying to report inventory without creating distortions in at least one key financial statement.

Consider an example in which we buy 1 unit of inventory on January 2 for $10 and another unit of inventory on December 30 for $20. On December 31, we sell a unit for $30. What happens to the financial statements if we are using the FIFO method of inventory tracking? The FIFO method means that the inventory that is first in is the inventory that is first out. The January 2 purchase was the first one in, so the cost of the unit sold is $10 and the cost of the unit remaining on hand is $20. What would it cost to buy a unit of inventory near year end? Well, we bought one on December 30 for $20, so the balance sheet seems pretty accurate.

However, consider the income statement under FIFO. We presumably sold the first in, which cost $10, for a selling price of $30, leaving us with a $20 profit. Is that a good indication of the profit we could currently earn from the purchase and sale of a unit of inventory? Not really. At year end we could have bought a unit for $20 and sold it for $30, leaving a profit of only $10. Thus, during periods of rising prices, the FIFO method does not give users of financial statements a current picture of the profit opportunities facing the organization.

We do not have that problem with LIFO. Under LIFO, the last in is the first out, which means that we sold the unit that was purchased on December 30. That unit had cost us $20, and by selling it for $30 we realize a profit of $10. When we tell our stockholders that our profit was $10, we are giving them a reasonably current picture of the profit we can currently make by buying and selling a unit.

Unfortunately this gives rise to another problem. Under LIFO, we have sold the unit that cost $20, so we must have held onto the unit that cost $10. Is it true that we could currently go out and buy more inventory for $10 a unit? No, by year end the price we paid was already up to $20. So, under LIFO, the value of inventory on the balance sheet is understated.

There is no readily available solution to this problem. The weighted average method simply leaves both the balance sheet and income statements somewhat out of whack, instead of causing a somewhat bigger problem with respect to one or the other, as results under LIFO and FIFO. In the face of this problem, for-profit organizations have shifted to LIFO for a very simple reason: to save taxes.

Let's take a second to consider the implication of our example. If we use a FIFO system during inflationary periods, we report a pretax profit of $20 because we have sold a unit that cost $10 for $30. Under LIFO, we report a pretax profit of only $10 because we have sold a unit that cost $20 for $30. Therefore, by being on the LIFO system, we can reduce our tax payments. Are the tax savings worth the fact that we will be reporting lowered profits on our financial statements? Absolutely. If we can lower our taxes by using allowable GAAP, we should take advantage of that opportunity.

However, it gets even better. Suppose we purchase a unit on January 2 for $10. On July 1 we sell that unit. On December 30 we buy a unit for $20. Which unit did we sell? You probably think we sold the unit we paid $10 for. However, you are now entering the accountant's world of make-believe.

Inventory accounting make-believe is played this way. Under FIFO we record $10 of expense and $20 of inventory as an asset. But under LIFO we record $20 of expense on the income statement and $10 as an asset on the balance sheet! That implies that we sold the unit we acquired on December 30, even though the sale took place 6 months earlier.

The accountant knows that obviously this can't physically be so. But that's okay. We'll just make believe that that's what happened. Under LIFO there is no need for us to actually move our inventories on a LIFO basis. We don't have to throw our conveyor belt into reverse, or keep milk on hand until it turns sour. If our product is dated, there is no need to feel we can't be on a LIFO system because we can't afford to keep stock on hand past the expiration date.

The organization on LIFO can continue to behave all year long as if it were on FIFO. Your managers should continue to make their product decisions based on the current cost of inventory items—and that usually requires a FIFO-type approach. However, your accountant at year end makes adjustments to your financial records to calculate your income as if you were consuming your inventory on a LIFO basis.

Assume the following:

Beginning Inventory	$ 0
January 3, Purchase 1 Unit @	$ 10
July 1, Sell 1 Unit @	$ 30
December 1, Purchase 1 Unit @	$ 20

Under either method, the first unit purchased was physically shipped and the second unit purchased was physically on hand at the end of the year. From a standpoint of physical movement of goods, the FIFO income statement tells the truth. However, by making believe that we shipped a unit that we hadn't even received by the shipping date, we can report a higher cost of goods used expense, and therefore report a lower profit and pay the government less tax.

The LIFO Conformity Rule

When we talked about depreciation in Chapter 9, we noted that we could have our cake and eat it too. We could tell our stockholders what a good year we had, but we could also tell the government how miserable things had really been. This is not true with LIFO. The government requires that the organization use the same method of inventory reporting to stockholders as it uses to report to the government.

Who Shouldn't Use LIFO

Many, many organizations could benefit from LIFO, but there are some that would not. LIFO is not necessarily advantageous if the cost of your inventory is highly uncertain, and veers downward as often as upward. For organizations dealing in commodities, WA remains a better bet. Organizations whose inventory costs are actually falling (computer chips, for example) will have lower taxes by staying on FIFO.

What if your inventory contains some items with rising cost and some items with falling cost? If you segment the inventory adequately, it is possible to report some of your inventory using one method and some of it based on another method.

LIFO Liquidations

The lower tax paid by an organization on LIFO is caused by reporting to the government that the most recent, high-priced purchases were sold while the old, low-cost items were kept. If we ever liquidate our inventory and sell everything we have, we incur a high profit on the sale of those low-cost items and have to pay back the taxes we would have paid had we been on FIFO all along. However, in the meantime we have had an interest-free loan from the government. If our year-end inventory is always at least as big as the beginning inventory, we will never have that problem and we will never have to repay those extra taxes to the government.

How about not-for-profit health care organizations? Can we assume that taxes make LIFO beneficial to for-profit organizations, but that not-for-profit health care organizations will stick with FIFO? No. If it turns out that any of your revenue results from a reimbursement of your costs, LIFO will help you. Suppose that a foundation offers to pay for the care for some group of disadvantaged patients. However, since they don't feel you should profit from treating those patients, the foundation agrees to just reimburse the cost of care. If you are using FIFO, the inventory you consume in treating those patients will be reported at a lower cost than if you use LIFO. So it turns out that revenue maximization would lead even not-for-profit health care organizations to use LIFO for their inventory cost-flow assumptions.

KEY CONCEPTS

The Inventory Equation

Beginning Inventory (BI)	+	Units Purchased (P)	−	Units Sold (S)	=	Ending Inventory (EI)

Periodic versus perpetual inventory—Different methods for keeping track of how many units have been used and how many units are on hand.

> *Periodic*—Goods are counted periodically to determine the ending inventory. The number of units used is calculated using the inventory equation.
>
> *Perpetual*—The inventory balance is adjusted as each unit is used so that a perpetual record of how many units have been used and how many are on hand is maintained at all times.

Cost-flow assumptions—Inventory is valued at its cost. Therefore, it is necessary to know not only how many units were used and how many are left on hand, but specifically which were used and which are left. This determination is made via one of four different approaches.

Specific identification—We record and identify each unit as it is acquired or used.

First-in, First-out (FIFO)—We assume that the units acquired earlier are used before units acquired later.

Weighted average (WA)—We assume that all units are indistinguishable and assign a weighted average cost to each unit.

Last-in, First-out (LIFO)—We assume that the last units acquired are the first ones used, even if this implies use of a unit prior to its acquisition. During periods of inflation there are tax savings associated with LIFO.

TEST YOUR KNOWLEDGE

See www.jbpub.com/catalog/0763726753/supplements.htm.

CHAPTER 11

An Even Closer Look
at Financial Statements

Earlier, we examined the source of financial statements. We discussed the basic definitions of assets, liabilities, net assets, revenues, and expenses. We traced through a variety of journal entries, and saw how ledger balances can be used to derive key financial statements. To understand financial information, it is vital to have an understanding of where this information comes from.

We now turn our attention to trying to get as much useful information as possible from a set of financial statements. There are a variety of reasons for wanting to be able to do this. First and foremost is to enable us to manage our organization better. Second, we want to be able to review the financial statements of close competitors to evaluate our performance as compared to theirs. Third, we may want to evaluate the financial statements of an organization in which we wish to invest. Fourth, we want to evaluate the financial statements of organizations we are considering extending credit to.

We may be looking for different types of information in each case. Before investing in an organization, we wish to know about its potential profitability; before extending credit, we want to assess an organization's liquidity and solvency. The goal of financial statement analysis is to derive from financial statements the information needed to make informed decisions.

We do this primarily through examination of the notes that accompany the financial statements and through the use of a technique called *ratio analysis*. Generally accepted accounting principles (GAAP), in recognition of many of the limitations of financial numbers generated by accounting systems, require that clarifying notes accompany financial statements. The information contained in these notes may be more relevant and important than the basic statements themselves. *Ratio analysis* is a method for examining the numbers contained in financial statements to see if there are relationships among the numbers that can provide us with useful information.

Chapter 12 focuses on the notes to the financial statements and Chapter 13 discusses ratio analysis. In the remainder of this chapter, we present a hypothetical set of financial statements to use as a basis for discussion.

THE BALANCE SHEET

Table 11-1 presents the balance sheet for the hypothetical Community Hospital (CH) that is the subject of our analysis. Information is provided for 2 years. In recognition of the

Table 11-1

Community Hospital
Statement of Financial Position
As of December 31, 2007 and December 31, 2006 (in '000)

	2007	2006
ASSETS		
Current Assets		
Cash	$ 16,000	$ 14,000
Marketable Securities	24,000	18,000
Accounts Receivables, Net	44,000	60,000
Inventory	98,000	80,000
Prepaid Expenses	6,000	4,000
Total Current Assets	$ 188,000	$ 176,000
Fixed Assets		
Buildings and Equipment	$ 300,000	$ 240,000
Less Accumulated Depreciation	80,000	60,000
Net Buildings and Equipment	$ 220,000	$ 180,000
Land	100,000	100,000
Total Fixed Assets	$ 320,000	$ 280,000
Goodwill	$ 90,000	$ 100,000
TOTAL ASSETS	$ 598,000	$ 556,000
	2007	2006
LIABILITIES & NET ASSETS		
Current Liabilities		
Wages Payable	$ 6,000	$ 4,000
Accounts Payable	58,000	50,000
Unearned Revenue	30,000	24,000
Total Current Liabilities	$ 94,000	$ 78,000
Long-Term Liabilities		
Mortgage Payable	$ 90,000	$ 100,000
Bond Payable	200,000	200,000
Other	78,000	70,000
Total Long-Term Liabilities	$ 368,000	$ 370,000
Net Assets		
Unrestricted	$ 66,000	$ 38,000
Temporarily Restricted	20,000	20,000
Permanently Restricted	50,000	50,000
Total Net Assets	$ 136,000	$ 108,000
TOTAL LIABILITIES & NET ASSETS	$ 598,000	$ 556,000

The accompanying notes are an integral part of these statements.

fact that information in a vacuum is not very useful, accountants generally provide comparative data. In the case of CH, the financial statements present the current fiscal year ending December 31, 2007, and the previous fiscal year ended December 31, 2006. Many financial reports contain the current year and the 2 previous years for comparison.

All the numbers on the CH statements are rounded to the nearest million dollars. You should be very careful to note that the title of the financial statement includes a note telling the reader that the figures are presented without three zeros or in thousands. This is what is meant at the end of the title by the words "in '000." In other words, the $16,000 listed for cash is really $16,000,000. This is common practice for large organizations, and accountants often round numbers to thousands or in some cases millions. Although this may seem like the accountant is not being very accurate, you must remember accounting and especially audited accounting statements are not expected to be perfectly accurate. Rounding the figures is a result of the the materiality principle discussed earlier in this book. Additionally, rounding makes the statements much easier to read.

Current Assets

The first assets listed on the balance sheet are the *current assets*. These are the most liquid of the organization's resources. The current assets are presented on the balance sheet in order of liquidity. *Cash*, the most readily available asset for use in meeting obligations as they become due, is listed first. Cash includes amounts on deposit in checking and savings accounts as well as cash on hand. The next item is *marketable securities* that are intended to be liquidated in the near term. They can be converted to cash in

a matter of a few days. Marketable securities that the organization intends to hold as long-term investments shouldn't be listed with current assets, but instead under a long-term investment category, after fixed assets.

The next current asset listed is *accounts receivable, net*. It is usually the case that we do not expect to collect all of the money that is due us from all of our patients and insurers. Some of it will become bad debts. As discussed in Chapter 2, there are many different third-party payers and payment mechanisms. "Accounts receivables, net" represents gross charges less an allowance for bad debts and also less the various contractual allowances established with those third-party payers. For example, suppose that CH delivered health care services during the year for which the charges were $100,000. CH had $20,000 of contractual allowances, bringing the receivable down to $80,000. In addition, there was $20,000 worth of patient co-payments. Historically, 10% of all co-payments are never collected for a variety of reasons. Sometimes the patient moves away. Sometimes the patient just decides not to pay his or her bill. Sometimes CH hasn't recorded the correct address information and can't find the patient. CH therefore takes a bad debt allowance of $2,000 (10% of $20,000), bringing the net receivable down to $78,000.

Charges	$ 100,000
Contractual Allowance	(20,000)
Allowance for Bad Debt	(2,000)
Accounts Receivable, net	$ 78,000

Inventory is generally listed on the balance sheet after receivables. This is because it is less liquid than receivables. The reason for this is that inventory is used to provide patient care services. Once those services have been provided, we can issue bills to patients, and accounts receivables arise. So clearly, inventory takes longer to convert to cash than receivables, because it has not yet been used to provide services. *Prepaid expenses* are grouped with current assets even though they do not usually generate any cash to use for paying current liabilities. Rather we expect them to be used up within the coming year. Prepaid expenses generally include items such as prepaid rent or insurance.

Health insurance companies often have prepaid expenses on their balance sheets. Typically, these represent capitated arrangements with providers. The insurance company pays a provider up-front for a certain set of services to be provided to a specific group of patients. When the insurance company pays the provider it has two entries on its ledger; cash goes down and the asset called prepaid insurance goes up. Conceptually, the health insurance company is trading one asset (cash) for another (the claim to services). As time goes by, the claim on services goes down and the insurance company must recognize the expense of these services.

In this example, the provider's balance sheet records mirror image entries. The provider receives the cash and has an obligation to provide health care services. In this case, cash goes up and the provider creates a liability called *unearned* or *deferred revenue*. As time goes by, and the provider has earned the revenue, the liability (unearned revenue) is reduced and insurance revenue is recognized.

Long-Term Assets

All assets the organization has that are not current assets fall into the general category of long-term assets. Prominent among the long-term assets are fixed assets, which include the property, plant, and equipment used to process or produce the organization's product or service. A variety of other long-term assets may also appear on the balance sheet. There would be a category for investments if we had marketable securities that we anticipated keeping for longer than 1 year.

In the case of CH, there is an asset called *goodwill*, an intangible asset that may arise through the acquisition of another organization (perhaps a physician practice). Most organizations have some goodwill: they have customer loyalty and a good relationship with their suppliers. However, goodwill is an intangible asset that accountants usually leave off the balance sheet because of the difficulty in measuring it. When one organization takes over another, if it pays more for the organization it is acquiring than can reasonably be assigned as the fair market value of the specific identifiable assets that it is buying, then the excess is recorded on the balance sheet of the acquiring organization as goodwill. This follows the accountant's philosophy that people are not fools. If we pay more for an organization than its other assets are worth, then there is a presumption that the various intangibles we are acquiring that can't be directly valued must be worth at least the excess amount we paid.

Liabilities

The organization's current *liabilities* are those that exist at the balance sheet date, which have to be paid in the next operating cycle—usually considered to be 1 year. Common current liabilities include wages payable, accounts payable, and in for-profit organizations, taxes payable. The taxes payable include only the portion to be paid in the near term, not the taxes that have been deferred more than 1 year beyond the balance sheet date.

Long-term liabilities include any recorded liabilities that are not current liabilities.

There may be a variety of commitments that the organization has made that will not be included with the liabilities. For example, if the organization has operating leases, they do not appear on the balance sheet, even though they may legally obligate the organization to make large payments into the future. The notes to the financial statements are especially important in disclosing material commitments.

Net Assets and Stockholders' Equity

As discussed earlier, *Net Assets* represents the difference between assets and liabilities. In not-for-profit organizations this can be thought of as the community's claim on the assets of the organization. This is conceptually similar to stockholders' equity in for-profit organizations. *Stockholders' equity* represents the outstanding claim that stockholders have on the organization. In most instances, the organization does not have an amount of cash equivalent to net assets or stockholders' equity. Rather, profits that have been earned over time, and that belong to the community or to the stockholders, have been reinvested in the organization in the form of equipment or other items to help the organization meet its mission and earn additional profits in the future.

In our CH example, net assets has three components: unrestricted, temporarily restricted, and permanently restricted. *Unrestricted net assets* represent an unfettered claim on a share of the organization's assets. To the extent that there are unrestricted net assets, the organization has an ability to make decisions about how to use an equivalent amount of the organization's assets.

Temporarily restricted net assets are typically restricted for a certain period of time or until a certain event occurs. These net assets usually arise as the result of either a grant or a donation that comes with strings attached. Suppose that a foundation offers CH a $100,000 research grant to participate in a national research study. However, the money must all be used on expenses related to that study. When CH receives the money, cash goes up. Liabilities don't change because the money is a grant; it is not owed back to the Foundation. On the other hand, CH is not free to do whatever they would like with that money. By treating the $100,000 as a temporarily restricted net asset, it ensures that everyone knows that the organization is not free to use that money however it would like. Similarly, when donors restrict their donations to a specific purpose or a specific time period for use, temporarily restricted net assets help to keep everything clear. Once the restrictions have been met, the temporarily restricted net assets become unrestricted.

Permanently restricted net assets are just that, permanently restricted as to their use. Generally they arise when donors are trying to provide for an endowment. Such endowments are invested and their earnings can be used by the organization. If the donor doesn't give specific conditions on a permanently restricted gift, beyond the permanent restriction, then the earnings can be used for any reasonable purpose such as operations or capital asset acquisitions. However, sometimes donors specify that the earnings from the endowment must be used for a particular purpose. In that case, as money is earned on the endowment investment, those earnings immediately become temporarily restricted net assets. They remain temporarily restricted until they are used in the manner specified by the donor.

If CH were a publicly traded for-profit health care organization, the balance sheet would contain a stockholders' equity section (instead of net assets) similar to Table 11-2.

The stockholders' equity section of the balance sheet contains a number of elements. Instead of simply having contributed capital and retained earnings, there are a number of separate items that comprise contributed capital. In addition, there is a distinction between amounts paid representing *par value* and *amounts in excess of par*. Par value is a new term that is discussed in this section.

In our example, there are two general classes of stock. There is common stock and preferred stock. *Common stock* is a traditional means of obtaining capital in many for-profit organizations. Investors purchase shares of the organization's assets in the form of stock. As stockholders, the investors become the owners of the organization and have the right to elect a board of directors and have a right to a share of any profit distributions. *Preferred stock* is a bit different. In this case, the organization generates capital by selling ownership rights (stock) with predetermined dividend payments. The specifics of common and preferred stock are discussed in more detail in Chapter 16.

Par value is a legal concept. In many states, organizations are required to set an arbitrary amount as the par value of their stock. One of the primary reasons many organizations incorporate is to achieve a limited liability for their owners. *Limited liability*

assumes that the corporation's stock was originally issued for at least its par value. If stock is issued below the par value—let's say that $10 par value stock is issued for $7—then the owner could be liable for the difference between the issue price and the par value should the organization go bankrupt. Given that situation, the par value of the corporation's stock is generally set low enough so that all stock is issued for at least the par value. Par value is an arbitrary value set by the organization.

There is no connection between the par value and any underlying value of the organization. There is no reason to believe that the arbitrarily selected par value is a good measure of what a share of stock is worth. In fact, because most organizations are very careful to set par low enough so that there is no extra liability for the corporation's owners, par value has become almost meaningless. Therefore, some states now allow corporations to issue stock without assigning a par value (called no par stock).

From an accounting perspective, we wish to be able to show the user of financial statements whether there is some potential additional liability to the stockholders. To accomplish this, the accountant has one account to show amounts received for stock up to the par value amount. Anything paid

Table 11-2	Stockholders' Equity Component of Statement of Financial Position As of December 31, 2007 and December 31, 2006 (in '000)		
		2007	**2006**
Stockholders' Equity			
Common Stock, $1 Par, 1000 Shares		$ 1,000	$ 1,000
Common Stock-Excess over Par		24,000	24,000
Preferred Stock, 10%, $100 Par, 100 Shares		10,000	10,000
Retained Earnings		101,000	73,000
Total Stockholders' Equity		$ 136,000	$ 108,000

above par for any share goes into a separate account with a name such as "excess paid over par" or "additional paid-in capital."

In our example, we see that CH has 1,000 shares of $1 par value common stock. The balance in the common stock par account is $1,000, meaning that all 1,000 shares were issued for at least $1 each, the par value. There are 100 shares of $100 par value preferred stock and the balance in the preferred stock par account is $10,000, indicating that each of the 100 shares was issued for at least $100. Therefore, we know that the stockholders have limited liability. They can lose everything they've paid for their stock, but if the organization goes bankrupt, creditors cannot attempt to collect additional amounts from the stockholders personally.

As is quite commonly the case, the stockholders in our example have paid more than the par value for at least some of the stock issued by the corporation. The common stock excess over par account has a balance of $24,000. Together with the $1,000 in the common stock par account, this indicates the investors paid $25,000 (or gave the firm resources worth $25,000) for 1,000 shares of stock. On average, investors paid $25 per share for the common stock. There is no excess over par account for the preferred stock. Therefore, we know that the preferred stockholders each paid exactly $100 per share for the preferred stock at the time it was issued.

The preferred stock is referred to as 10%, $100 par stock, indicating that the annual dividend rate on the preferred stock is 10% of the $100 par value. Each preferred share must receive a $10 dividend before the organization can pay any dividend to the common stock shareholders.

The retained earnings, as discussed previously, represent the profits that the organization earned during its existence that have not been distributed to the stockholders as dividends, and therefore have been retained in the organization. Remember that this category, like the others on the liability and owners' equity side of the balance sheet, represents claims on assets. There is no pool of money making up the retained earnings. Rather, the profits earned over the years and retained in the organization have likely been invested in a variety of fixed and current assets.

Excel Template

You may use Template 8 to prepare a balance sheet for your organization. The template is on the Web at www.jbpub.com.

STATEMENT OF OPERATIONS

As discussed earlier, the *statement of operations* (often referred to as the *income statement*) is a flow statement. Its primary purpose is to show the flow of revenues (increases in wealth) and expenses (decreases in wealth) for the organization over a given period of time. Table 11-3 shows the statement of operations for CH. As is the case with most health care organizations, CH derives the vast majority of its revenues from patient services. As you can see, they also have a reasonable amount of premium revenue (this is often based on capitated per member per month charges). The statement of operations is divided into two main sections. On top, revenues and expenses are listed and together yield the net gain or loss from operations (often listed as Excess of Revenues over Expenses). Below the operating section are changes in net assets that are not from operating activities. These "below-the-line" changes must be shown to be able to link the beginning net asset value with the ending net asset value on the balance sheet. The below-the-line changes may include items such as contributions,

Table 11-3

Community Hospital
Statement of Operations
For the Years Ended December 31, 2007 and December 31, 2006 (in '000)

	2007	2006
Revenues		
Net Patient Services Revenue	$ 180,000	$ 159,000
Premium Revenue	29,000	20,000
Other Operating Revenue	15,000	12,000
Total Revenues From Operations	$ 224,000	$ 191,000
Expenses		
Salaries and Benefits	$ 75,000	$ 68,000
Medical Supplies and Drugs	95,000	87,000
Insurance	15,000	12,000
Depreciation	20,000	16,000
Interest	2,000	3,000
Provision for Bad Debts	5,000	3,000
Total Expenses From Operations	$ 212,000	$ 189,000
Excess of Revenues over Expenses	$ 12,000	$ 2,000
Unrestricted Contributions	56,000	40,000
Transfers to Parent	(40,000)	(35,000)
Increase/(Decrease) in Unrestricted Net Assets	$ 28,000	$ 7,000

transfers to or from a parent organization, or other non-operating transactions.

To understand the link between the statement of operations and the balance sheet all one has to do is look at the ending unrestricted net asset balance from Table 11-1. For the year ended 2006, CH had unrestricted net assets of $38,000. The following year, CH ended with unrestricted net assets on the balance sheet of $66,000. This represents a change of $28,000 for the 2007 fiscal year. This change is shown on the bottom of the statement of operations (Table 11-3). In reality, the statement of operations is nothing more than a listing of all the changes that affect the net assets. It is organized into an operating section that includes the or-

ganizations revenues and expenses and a non-operating section that captures other changes to net assets.

In publicly traded for-profit health care organizations, the statement of operations must also include earnings per share data. The earnings per share data is shown below all the information described above. Table 11-4 shows an example of this portion of a statement of operations. In Table 11-4, we use a Net Income number that is different from the Increase in Unrestricted Net Assets that we saw in Table 11-3. These numbers are normally the same, but in this example we changed the net income number so that we can demonstrate the impact of dividends on the retained earnings balance. The num-

Table 11-4	Earnings Per Share Component of Statement of Operations For the Years Ended December 31, 2007 and December 31, 2006 (in '000)			
		2007		**2006**
Net Income		$ 33,000		$ 10,000
Earnings Per Share Common	$ 32.00		$ 9.00	
Less Dividends 2007 and 2006		5,000		3,000
Addition to Retained Earnings		$ 28,000		$ 7,000
Retained Earnings January 1, 2006 and 2005		73,000		66,000
Retained Earnings December 31, 2007 and 2006		$ 101,000		$ 73,000

bers presented in Table 11-4 match the retained earnings and stockholder's equity shown in Table 11-2.

The line following Net Income in Table 11-4 contains earnings per share data. GAAP require inclusion of information on a per-share basis for common stock. It is felt that this type of information may be more relevant than net income for many users of financial information. Consider an individual who owns 100 shares of common stock of a large corporation. The corporation reports that its profits have risen from $25,000,000 to $30,000,000. On the surface, we would presume that the stockholder is better off this year. What if, however, during the year the corporation issued additional shares of stock, thereby creating additional owners. Although total profits have risen $5,000,000 or 20%, because of the additional share of stock outstanding, investors find that their share of earnings increased by less than 20%. In fact, it is quite possible that the profits attributable to each individual share may have fallen, even though the total profit for the corporation has increased.

Table 11-4 begins with Net Income. Note that for-profit organizations use *Net Income*

on their operating statement rather than increase or decrease in net assets, which is used by not-for-profit organizations; conceptually they are the same. One of the main reasons for the difference in terminology is that not-for-profit organizations are reluctant to give the image of earning profits or income. They feel the public, and donors especially, won't understand that even not-for-profit organizations need to be profitable to be able to meet their mission.

Using the same stock information we used in Table 11-2, we see that although there are 1,000 shares of common stock and the net income was $33,000, the earnings or income (the two terms are used interchangeably) per share is $32.00, rather than the expected $33.00. This is because $1,000 has to be paid as a 10% dividend to the preferred shareholders. This portion of the income of the organization doesn't belong to the common shareholders. The remaining $32,000 does.

Looking at Table 11-2, we see that the balance in the common and preferred stock accounts didn't change during the year. However, the balance in retained earnings did change. The change in retained earnings on the balance sheet is mapped out at the bottom of Table 11-4. The beginning balance in Retained Earnings is combined with this year's addition to retained earnings to yield the end of year Retained Earnings listed on the balance sheet. This is the same tie between the balance sheet and statement of operations we discussed earlier with respect to unrestricted net assets.

Excel Template

You may use Template 9 to prepare a Statement of Operations for your organization. The template is on the Web at www.jbpub.com

---

STATEMENT OF CASH FLOWS

The statement of cash flows focuses on financial rather than operating aspects of the organization. Where did the money come from and how did the organization spend it? Whereas the major concern of the income statement is profitability, the statement of cash flows is very concerned with viability. Is the organization generating and will it generate enough cash to meet both short-term and long-term obligations?

There are two methods currently used for presenting the statement of cash flows: the direct method and the indirect method. In Chapter 4 we presented a simple direct method layout of the cash flow statement (see Table 4-3). As you may recall, the statement lists all the sources and uses of cash and organizes these into three categories: operating activities, investing activities, and financing activities. The main difference between the direct and indirect methods of laying out the statement is in the operating activities section of the statement.

Cash flow from operations is a focal point because it provides information on whether the routine operating activities of the organization generate cash, or require a cash infusion. If the operating activities generate a surplus of cash, the organization is more financially stable and viable than if they consume more cash than they generate. This does not mean that negative cash from operating activities is bad. It may be indicative of a growing, profitable organization that is expanding inventories and receivables as it grows. However, it does provide a note of caution. Overly rapid expansion, without other adequate cash sources, can cause some financial failure. Table 11-5 shows the Statement of Cash Flows for CH using the direct method.

Table 11-6 shows the same information as it would be displayed using the indirect method. Instead of a straight listing of cash flow transactions, the indirect method starts with the increase in unrestricted net assets from the last line of the operating statement and makes adjustments to reconcile to actual cash flow. It is important to remember that under accrual accounting revenues and expenses are not the same thing as cash inflows and cash outflows. The operating statement reports revenues and expenses. The cash flow statement reports cash inflows and cash outflows.

The cash flows from operating activities are first approximated by the net income or change in unrestricted net assets of the organization. Revenue activities are generally generators of cash, and expenses generally consume cash. That is not always the case, however, and a number of adjustments are needed. First of all, there are certain expenses that do not consume cash. In Table 11-6, note that several expenses are added to the increase in net assets. Depreciation reflects a current year expense for a portion of fixed assets that are being used up during the year. These assets were mostly purchased in earlier years, and paid for at that time. The operating statement charges part of

Table 11-5

Community Hospital
Statement of Cash Flows (Direct Method)
For the Years Ended December 31, 2007 and December 31, 2006 (in '000)

	2007	2006
Cash Flows From Operating Activities		
Collections	$ 237,000	$ 198,000
Payments to Suppliers	(105,000)	(96,000)
Payments to Employees	(60,000)	(75,000)
Insurance Payments	(16,000)	(14,000)
Interest Payments	(2,000)	(3,000)
Net Cash From Operating Activities	$ 54,000	$ 10,000
Cash Flow From Investing Activities		
Increase in Marketable Securities	$ (6,000)	
Sale of Fixed Assets	0	$ 2,000
Purchase of New Equipment	(60,000)	
Net Cash (Used for)/From Investing Activities	$ (66,000)	$ 2,000
Cash Flow From Financing Activities		
Payment of Mortgage Principal	$ (10,000)	$ (10,000)
Transfers to Parent	(40,000)	(40,000)
Additional Long-term Debt	8,000	6,000
Unrestricted Contributions	56,000	40,000
Net Cash (Used for)/From Financing Activities	$ 14,000	$ (4,000)
Net Increase/(Decrease) in Cash	$ 2,000	$ 8,000
Cash, Beginning of Year	14,000	6,000
Cash, End of Year	$ 16,000	$ 14,000

their cost as an expense in the current year. However, that does not require any cash. Similarly, a reduction in the value of goodwill (called *impairment of goodwill*) often occurs only years after payment was made to acquire that goodwill. Therefore, the change in net assets or net income is an imperfect measure of cash flow. It treats all expenses as if they consumed cash. Because depreciation and impairment do not consume cash, they are added back. To the extent that cash was actually spent this year on fixed asset pur-

chases, it shows up in the investing activity portion of the statement of cash flows.

In addition to these expense items, there are a variety of other activities related to operations that consume or provide cash, but are not adequately approximated by the change in net assets. For example, when the organization purchases more inventory than it uses, the extra inventory is not an expense. Nevertheless, we must pay for it, so there is a cash flow. Increases in inventory must therefore be subtracted to show that they consume

Table 11-6

Community Hospital
Statement of Cash Flows (In-Direct Method)
For the Years Ended December 31, 2007 and December 31, 2006 (in '000)

	2007	2006
Cash Flows From Operating Activities		
Increase in Unrestricted Net Assets	$ 12,000	$ 2,000
Add Expenses Not Requiring Cash:		
Depreciation	20,000	16,000
Impairment of Goodwill	10,000	0
Other Adjustments:		
Add Reduction in Accounts Receivable	16,000	$ 2,000
Add Increase in Wages Payable	2,000	0
Add Increase in Accounts Payable	8,000	3,000
Add Increase in Unearned Revenue	6,000	0
Subtract Decrease in Accounts Payable	0	(6,000)
Subtract Increase in Inventory	(18,000)	(7,000)
Subtract Increase in Prepaid Expenses	(2,000)	0
Net Cash (Used for)/From Investing Activities	$ 54,000	$ 10,000
Cash Flows From Investing Activties		
Increase in Marketable Securities	$ (6,000)	
Sale of Fixed Assets	0	$ 2,000
Purchase of New Equipment	(60,000)	
Net Cash (Used for)/From Investing Activities	$ (66,000)	$ 2,000
Cash Flows From Financing Activities		
Payment of Mortgage Principal	$ (10,000)	$ (10,000)
Transfers to Parent	(40,000)	(40,000)
Additional Long-term Debt	8,000	6,000
Unrestricted Contributions	56,000	40,000
Net Cash From/(Used for) Financing Activities	$ 14,000	$ (4,000)
Net Increase/(Decrease) in Cash	$ 2,000	$ 8,000
Cash, Beginning of Year	14,000	6,000
Cash, End of Year	$ 16,000	$ 14,000

cash. On the other hand, if wages payable increase, that indicates that less cash was currently paid than we would expect based on the labor expenses we had for the year.

These adjustments can become complicated. However, for the nonfinancial manager it is not necessary to be able to make the various adjustments. Nonfinancial managers should focus on interpretation of the numbers. It is more important to be aware of the fact that these components show us what is affecting cash from operating activities. For instance, increases in accounts receivable require a subtraction from the increase in net assets. This is because net income assumes that all revenues have been received. If accounts receivable are rising, the organization is not collecting all of its revenues from the current year. If we note a large increase in accounts receivable, it warns the managers that perhaps greater collections efforts are in order.

The second part of the statement of cash flows is cash from investing activities. We note here that CH increased its marketable securities, using $6,000 of cash, and purchased new equipment for $60,000. In the prior year, some equipment was sold.

The third section of the statement of cash flows is from financing activities. CH had one cash inflow during the year in the form of $8,000 worth of additional long-term debt. The other financing activities include payment of principal on an existing mortgage in the amount of $10,000 and a $40,000 transfer of cash to CH's parent organization. Many health care organizations are part of larger health care systems (or corporations). As part of the "system" arrangement, funds often flow to the parent as well as flowing from the parent.

Combining the cash flows from operating, investing, and financing activities yields the net increase or decrease in cash for the year. Added to the cash balance at the beginning of the year, this provides the cash balance at the end of the year. This is the same balance as that appearing on the balance sheet (Table 11-1).

For CH the final cash balance has not been varying substantially. At the end of 2007 the balance is $16,000. The prior year

it was $14,000. More important than the stability in the closing balance each year is the fact that the investments made by CH are being financed from operating activities. Not only are operations generating a positive cash flow, but further this cash flow is generally sufficient, or nearly sufficient, to cover the organization's investing and financing needs.

Right now, CH is relatively stable. It is growing and profitable, has twice as much in current assets as current liabilities, and has sustained its cash balance. On the other hand, as growth continues it must carefully monitor this statement. Increases in fixed assets, inventory, and receivables that normally accompany growth may prevent the organization from remaining in balance. Managers should consider whether the cash being generated from activities is sufficient to sustain planned growth. If not, they should start to plan for additional increases in long-term debt. A specific focus on the statement of cash flows can be a tremendous aid to management in preparing an orderly approach to meeting the financial needs of the organization.

Excel Template

You may use Template 10 to prepare a Statement of Cash Flows for your organization. The template is on the Web at www.jbpub.com.

THE NOTES TO THE FINANCIAL STATEMENTS

This chapter introduces you to the financial statements of CH. We discuss these statements in somewhat more detail than the statements we looked at in earlier chapters. However, no matter how closely you read the numbers in the financial statements nor how well you understand the detail presented on the financial statements, in themselves they are an inadequate picture of the organization.

The balance sheet, statement of operations, and statement of cash flows of an audited set of financial statements all refer the reader to the "notes" that follow or accompany the financial statements. Accounting is not a science. It is a set of rules containing numerous exceptions and complications. Financial analysis requires an understanding of what the organization's financial position really is and what the results of its operations and cash flows really were. It is vital that the user of financials not simply look to the total assets and net income to determine how well the organization has done. The notes that accompany the financial statements really are an integral part of the annual report. It is to those notes for CH that we turn in Chapter 12.

KEY CONCEPTS

Financial statement analysis—Techniques of analyzing financial statement information to find out as much about the organization's financial position and the results of its operations and its cash flows as possible. The focus is on the financial statements, the notes to the financial statements, and ratio analysis.

Par value—Legal concept related to limited liability of stockholders. There is no relationship between par value and a fair or correct value of the organization's stock.

Earnings per share—Rather than focus simply on net income or total earnings, GAAP require disclosure of the earnings available to common shareholders on a per-share basis.

TEST YOUR KNOWLEDGE

See www.jbpub.com/catalog/0763726753/supplements.htm.

CHAPTER 12

Notes to the Financial Statements: The Inside Story

The financial statements for Community Hospital (CH) tell a great deal about the organization. We have information about the organization's resources, obligations, net worth (net assets), profitability, and cash flows. Yet financial statements are extremely limited in their ability to convey information. Therefore, audited financial statements must be accompanied by a set of *notes*. These notes explain the organization's significant accounting policies and provide disclosure of other information not contained in the balance sheet, statement of operations, and statement of cash flows, but that is necessary for the statements to be a fair representation of the organization's financial position and the results of its operations.

This chapter presents a hypothetical set of notes for the financial statements of CH. We first present each note and then discuss it before moving on to the next note. This discussion is not exhaustive. Each organization has notes that apply to its own unique circumstances.

SIGNIFICANT ACCOUNTING POLICIES

The notes section generally begins with a statement of accounting policies. This is particularly important because of the alternative choices of accounting methods allowed, even within the constraints of generally accepted accounting principles (GAAP). In cases in which the organization has a choice of methods, that choice likely has an impact on both the balance sheet and the statement of operations and possibly on the statement of cash flows. The financial statement figures are not meaningful unless we know what choices the organization has made.

NOTE A: Significant Accounting Policies

1. *Net Patient Services Revenue—The Hospital has arrangements with third-party payers that provide for payments to the Hospital at amounts different from established rates.* Net patient services revenue *is recorded at the estimated net realizable amounts from patients and third-party payers.*

This note makes it clear that CH does not claim full charges as revenue. As described earlier in this book, health care organizations have a variety of payment systems. *Net patient service revenue* represents the actual amount that the hospital is entitled to collect for the services it has provided, after subtracting charity care, negotiated discounts, and other contractual allowances.

2. *Short-term investments—Short-term invest-*
   ments are stated at their fair market value.

CH has $24,000 of marketable securities at the end of fiscal year 2007 (see Table 11-1). Your expectation might well be that these securities cost CH $24,000 because that would correspond with the *cost* principle of accounting. However, objective market prices for stocks and bonds are available from many sources. We can determine the price at which identical securities were actually sold. Therefore, marketable securities are generally shown on the balance sheet at their fair market value.

3. *Inventories—Inventories are stated at cost,*
   not to exceed market. Cost is calculated
   using the last-in, first-out (LIFO) method.

Here the principle of recording at cost (based on objective evidence) conflicts with that of conservatism (adequate consideration of relevant risks). In this case, GAAP requires use of lower of cost or market value (LCM). If the market value exceeds cost, we use the cost. If the cost exceeds market value, we use the market value. Essentially, we are willing to value inventory below its cost, but not above it.

So inventories are stated using LCM because of the GAAP of conservatism. But how does CH measure the cost of its inventory? This note tells us that CH uses the LIFO method to determine inventory cost. LIFO/FIFO is a choice the organization is allowed under GAAP.

4. *Property, plant, and equipment—Property,*
   plant, and equipment are recorded at cost,
   less depreciation. Depreciation taken over
   the useful lives of plant and equipment is
   calculated on the straight-line basis.

For financial reporting, we have a fair degree of latitude in choosing a depreciation method. We could use a declining balance or sum-of-the-years' digits approach as an alternative to straight-line depreciation. For CH in 2007, operating costs included $20,000 of depreciation calculated on a straight-line basis. Suppose that the double-declining balance depreciation would have been $32,000, and that the sum-of-the-years' digits depreciation would have been $26,000.

The organization's reported net income can be greatly affected by the choice of accounting methods. Disclosure of choices, such as the inventory and depreciation methods used, provides users with a greater ability to understand the organization's financial situation.

5. *Income Taxes—Community Hospital is a*
   not-for-profit organization as described in
   Internal Revenue Code 501(c)(3) and re-
   lated income is exempt from federal in-
   come tax under Code Section 501(a).

Like many health care organizations, CH is a not-for-profit organization and therefore does not pay income tax. This note identifies the specific sections of the IRS code under which CH is claiming its tax-exempt status.

6. *Charity Care—The Hospital provides care*
   without charge to patients who meet cer-
   tain criteria under its charity care policy.
   Because the Hospital has no expectation
   or claim on payment in such cases, no rev-
   enue related to charity care is reported.

Many health care organizations provide charity care. In fact, the IRS code specifically speaks to the issue of not-for-profits giving back to the community as a justification for their favorable tax-exempt status. Because the organization has no up-front expectation of being paid for the services rendered under its charity care policy, it cannot claim any revenues related to these services. Often, readers of health care financial statements expect to see expenses related to charity care specifically highlighted on the statement of operations. In reality, the expenses related to providing charity care are included in the operating statement in the form of expenses such as wages and supplies. They are not, however, listed as a separate expense, nor are they listed as revenue.

7. *Temporarily and Permanently Restricted Net Assets—Temporarily restricted net assets have been limited by donors to a specific time period or until a specific event. Permanently restricted net assets have restrictions set by donors that must be maintained in perpetuity.*

As described earlier, the net assets of not-for-profit health care organizations like CH have three categories: unrestricted, temporarily restricted, and permanently restricted. This note outlines the definitions being used for temporarily restricted and permanently restricted net assets.

OTHER NOTES

In addition to a summary of accounting policies, the annual report contains other notes that provide additional disclosure of information needed for the financial statements to provide a fair representation of the financial position of the organization and the results of its operations.

NOTE B: Receivables

Receivables at December 31, 2007, including applicable allowances, were as follows:

Patient accounts	$ 72,000
Less allowances for:	
Contractual adjustments	(22,000)
Uncollectibles	(6,000)
Receivables, Net	$ 44,000

The note on receivables provides the reader with additional information on the relation-ship between charges and actual payments. Based on the information provided here, it is clear that the big difference between charges and net receivables is the contractual allowance. This note also allows the reader to track changes in uncollectables to see if this is becoming a larger problem over time.

NOTE C: Bonds Payable

At December 31, 2007, the schedule of required payments on Community Hospital's outstanding bonds consisted of the following:

Year Ending December 31	Principal	Interest	Total
2007	$ —	$ 2,000	$ 2,000
2008	—	2,000	2,000
2009	—	2,000	2,000
2010	—	2,000	2,000
2011	—	2,000	2,000
2012–2016	68,000	14,000	82,000
2017–2021	45,000	12,000	57,000
2022–2026	46,000	11,500	57,500
2027–2031	41,000	12,700	53,700
Total	$ 200,000	$ 60,200	$ 260,200

The balance sheet of CH lists three classes of long-term debt: mortgages, bonds, and other. The long-term debt schedule included in the notes provides detailed information on the upcoming bond payment obligations. As can be seen, CH has obligations that are stable for the next 5 years, through 2011. In the period 2012 to 2016, they have $68,000 in bonds that come due and cause their total payments for those years to jump from $2,000 to $82,000. In most cases, health care industry bonds require that only interest be paid during the life of the bond with a full principal payment at maturity. The large principal payment at maturity causes spikes in an organization's debt payment schedule. In many cases, bonds or portions of them are refinanced as they reach maturity.

NOTE D: Commitments, Contingencies, and Litigation

Community Hospital is involved in a number of legal proceedings and claims with various parties that arose in the normal course of business. In the opinion of management, the outcome of the legal proceedings and claims is not expected to have a material adverse affect on the financial position of the entity.

The organization is required to disclose any material obligations or other possible liabilities or litigations that are significant. Recall that a financial transaction is not recorded unless there has been exchange. The organization may have recently settled a malpractice suit, but not had any accounting transactions. If the settlement is material, disclosure is required.

NOTE E: Goodwill

The goodwill recorded on the balance sheet arose as a result of the acquisition of another organization for more than fair market value of the identifiable assets of the organization. It has been determined that due to permanent changes in market conditions, the goodwill has lost 10% of its value during 2007. Therefore, goodwill has been reduced from $100,000 to $90,000 on the balance sheet and a $10,000 expense has been charged.

When one organization acquires another for more than the value of the specific identifiable resources, the excess is grouped under the category of *goodwill.* It is very common for goodwill to arise when acquisitions occur. If the ongoing organization being ac-

quired was not worth more than its specific assets, the purchaser might simply buy similar assets rather than acquiring the organization. Many intangibles arise over an organization's life, such as reputation for quality products and creditworthiness. Goodwill remains as an asset on the balance sheet indefinitely under current GAAP. Goodwill is only reduced when there is a clear impairment to its value. At such time, the entire impairment is treated as a one-time reduction in the value of goodwill. This differs from tax treatment that allows for-profit organizations to deduct the cost of goodwill as an expense over a 15-year period.

SUMMARY

This chapter does not present an all-inclusive listing of required notes to the financial statements. Depending on the exact circumstance of different organizations, a wide variety of disclosures are required by GAAP and by requirements of the Securities and Exchange Commission. The most important learning issue in this chapter is not the information contained in the notes discussed. Rather, it is that the reader should have an awareness of the importance of the information that is contained in the notes to the financial statements.

The notes to the financial statements may at first seem both overwhelming and boring. They certainly do not make for light reading. You have to work through them slowly and carefully to understand the information that each note is trying to convey. Exactly which choices has the organization made, and what are the implications of each choice? Is the organization reliant on one key customer? If so, that fact would have to be disclosed somewhere in the notes. Can the organization use all of its cash, or does it have a "compensating balance" agreement with its bank that requires it to maintain a minimum balance? If the latter, the organization's liquidity is somewhat overstated in the balance sheet. Compensating balance arrangements must be disclosed. Are there securities outstanding, such as convertible bonds that can be converted into common stock? If so, then the organization's net income might have to be shared among more stockholders. Such potential dilution, if significant, is discussed in the notes.

We could continue with examples of the types of information relevant to creditors, investors, and internal management contained only in the notes to the financials. Not all notes are relevant to all readers. Some items are of more concern to employees than to stockholders. Some items help creditors more than internal managers. Whatever your purpose in using a financial report, the key is that the financial statements by themselves are incapable of telling the full story. To avoid being misled by the numbers, it is necessary to supplement the information in the statements with the information in the notes that accompany the statements.

KEY CONCEPTS

Significant accounting policies—Whenever GAAP allow an organization a choice in accounting methods, the organization must disclose the choice that it made. This allows the user of financial statements to better interpret the numbers, such as net income, contained in the financial statements.

Other notes—The organization must disclose any information that a user of the financial statements might need to have a fair representation of the organization's financial position and the results of its operations in accordance with GAAP. This information should be included in either the financial statements themselves or the notes that accompany the financial statements.

TEST YOUR KNOWLEDGE

See www.jbpub.com/catalog/0763726753/supplements.htm.

CHAPTER 13

Ratio Analysis: How Do We Compare to Other Health Care Organizations?

So, we have generated the financial statements, had them audited, and have fully read the notes that accompany the statements. With a full understanding of the financial statements and the types of transactions that generated them, we can begin to use the information to help assess the financial health of the organization.

One of the most widely used forms of financial analysis is the use of *ratios*. Ratios can provide information that is useful for comparing one health care organization to another (*benchmarking*). Ratios can provide the information that banks and lenders use to determine if our organization can take on more debt. They can also help internal management of an organization gain an awareness of their company's strengths and weaknesses. And, if we can find weaknesses, we can move to correct them before irreparable damage is done.

What is a ratio? Basically, a ratio is a comparison of any two numbers. In financial statement analysis, we compare numbers taken from the financial statements. For instance, if we want to know how much Community Hospital (CH) had in current assets as compared to current liabilities at the end of fiscal 2007, we could compare its

$188,000 in current assets (Table 13-1) to its $94,000 in current liabilities. Mathematically, we could state this as $188,000 divided by $94,000, which is equal to 2. This means that there are 2 dollars of current assets for every 1 dollar of current liabilities. This is referred to either as a ratio of 2 or a ratio of 2 to 1. This particular ratio is called the current ratio. In this chapter, we discuss many widely used ratios, but the discussion is not all inclusive.

Different sectors of the health care system may have different ratios that are commonly used. It is important to remember that a ratio is merely the combination of two numbers that together show a relationship that often provides more useful information than the two numbers separately. You should feel free to create your own ratios that help to show meaningful relationships for your organization.

BENCHMARKS FOR COMPARISON

Is the CH current ratio of 2 good or bad? Is it high enough? Is it too high? We don't want to have too little in the way of current assets, or we may have a liquidity crisis (that is, insufficient cash to pay our obligations as

Table 13-1

Community Hospital
Statement of Financial Position
As of December 31, 2007 and December 31, 2006 (in 000's)

ASSETS

	2007		2006	
Current Assets				
Cash	2.7%	$ 16,000	2.5%	$ 14,000
Marketable Securities	4.0%	24,000	3.2%	18,000
Accounts Receivables, Net	7.4%	44,000	10.8%	60,000
Inventory	16.4%	98,000	14.4%	80,000
Prepaid Expenses	1.0%	6,000	0.7%	4,000
Total Current Assets	31.4%	$188,000	31.7%	$176,000
Fixed Assets				
Buildings and Equipment	50.2%	$300,000	43.2%	$240,000
Less Accumulated Depreciation	13.4%	80,000	10.8%	60,000
Net Buildings and Equipment	36.8%	$220,000	32.4%	$180,000
Land	16.7%	100,000	18.0%	100,000
Total Fixed Assets	53.5%	$320,000	50.4%	$280,000
Goodwill	15.1%	$ 90,000	18.0%	$100,000
TOTAL ASSETS	100.0%	$598,000	100.0%	$556,000

LIABILITIES & NET ASSETS

	2007		2006	
Current Liabilities				
Wages Payable	1.0%	$ 6,000	0.7%	$ 4,000
Accounts Payable	9.7%	58,000	9.0%	50,000
Unearned Revenue	5.0%	30,000	4.3%	24,000
Total Current Liabilities	15.7%	$ 94,000	14.0%	$ 78,000
Long-Term Liabilities				
Mortgage Payable	15.1%	$ 90,000	18.0%	$100,000
Bond Payable	33.4%	200,000	36.0%	200,000
Other	13.0%	78,000	12.6%	70,000
Total Long-Term Liabilities	61.5%	$368,000	66.5%	$370,000
Total Liabilities	77.3%	$462,000	80.6%	$448,000
Net Assets				
Unrestricted	11.0%	$ 66,000	6.8%	$ 38,000
Temporarily Restricted	3.3%	20,000	3.6%	20,000
Permanently Restricted	8.4%	50,000	9.0%	50,000
Total Net Assets	22.7%	$136,000	19.4%	$108,000
TOTAL LIABILITIES & NET ASSETS	100.0%	$598,000	100.0%	$556,000

they become due. We don't want to have too much in the way of current assets because this implies that we are passing up profitable long-term investment opportunities. But there is no correct number for the current ratio. We can only assess the appropriateness of our ratios on the basis of some benchmark or other basis for comparison.

There are three principal benchmarks. The first is the organization's history. We always want to review the ratios for the organization this year, compared to what they were in the several previous years. This enables us to discover favorable or unfavorable trends that are developing gradually over time, as well as pointing up any numbers that have changed sharply in the space of time of just 1 year.

The second type of benchmark is to compare the organization to specific competitors. If the competitors are publicly held companies, we can obtain copies of their annual reports and compare each of our ratios with each of theirs. This approach is especially valuable for helping to pinpoint why your organization is doing particularly better or worse than a specific competitor. By finding where your ratios differ, you may determine what you are doing better or worse than the competition.

The third type of benchmark is industry-wide comparison. Many consulting firms and benchmarking specialists, such as Solucient, collect financial data, compute ratios, and publish the results. Not only are industry averages available, but the information is often broken down both by size of the organization and in a way that allows determination of relatively how far away from the norm you are.

For example, if your current ratio is 2, and the industry average is 2.4, is that a substantial discrepancy? Published industry data may show that 25% of the organizations

in the industry have a current ratio below 1.5. In this case, we may not be overly concerned that our ratio of 2.0 is too low. We are still well above the bottom quartile. On the other hand, what if only 25% of the health care organizations have a current ratio of less than 2.1? In this case, over three quarters of the organizations have a higher current ratio than we do. This might be a cause for some concern. At the very least, we might want to investigate why our ratio is particularly low, compared to others. Table 13-2 presents one page from the *SourceBook* by Solucient. This page provides information about hospital profit margins over a period of 5 years. In addition, it breaks the information down by size of hospital (number of beds), urban/rural status, and other major classifications.

There are five principal types of ratios that we examine in this chapter. They are (1) common size ratios; (2) liquidity ratios; (3) efficiency ratios; (4) solvency ratios; and (5) profitability ratios.

COMMON SIZE RATIOS

Common size ratios are used as a starting point in financial statement analysis. Suppose that we wished to compare our organization to another. We look to our cash balance and see that it is $10,000, whereas the other firm has cash of $5,000. Does this mean we have too much cash? Does the other organization have too little cash? Before we can even begin to consider such questions, we need more general information about the two organizations. Are we twice as big as the other organization? Are we smaller than the other organization? The amount of cash we need depends on the size of our operations compared to theirs. Comparing our cash to their cash does not create a very useful ratio.

Table 13-2 Sample National Comparison: Total Profit Margin

Percentile	1999			1998			1997			1996	1995
	75th	50th	25th	75th	50th	25th	75th	50th	25th	50th	50th
All Hospitals	7.40	3.17	(1.03)	8.36	4.11	0.02	9.61	5.32	1.42	5.03	5.06
25 to 99 beds	6.56	2.45	(1.75)	7.03	3.01	(1.13)	8.59	4.42	0.02	4.12	4.19
100 to 249 beds	8.50	3.85	(0.69)	9.30	4.66	0.48	10.40	5.99	2.14	5.65	5.69
250 to 399 beds	8.69	4.29	0.37	9.90	5.80	1.39	11.00	6.57	2.65	6.63	5.95
400 and over	6.16	2.76	0.14	8.42	4.94	1.23	9.46	6.24	2.93	5.31	5.68
Urban	7.83	3.13	(1.06)	8.80	4.30	0.07	9.61	5.30	1.42	5.10	5.03
25 to 99 beds	6.30	1.99	(2.77)	6.79	2.33	(2.29)	8.06	3.00	(1.47)	3.47	3.66
100 to 249 beds	8.58	3.39	(1.22)	8.87	4.26	0.06	9.79	5.39	1.43	5.08	4.95
250 to 399 beds	8.67	4.02	0.25	9.85	5.73	1.21	10.75	6.18	2.43	6.21	5.94
400 and over	6.03	2.75	0.14	8.29	4.92	1.18	9.36	6.11	2.91	5.27	5.67
Rural	7.05	3.21	(0.99)	7.79	3.90	(0.10)	9.63	5.36	1.42	4.97	5.14
25 to 99 beds	6.61	2.61	(1.40)	7.04	3.21	(0.91)	8.88	4.73	0.47	4.27	4.46
100 to 249 beds	8.31	4.70	1.28	10.52	5.87	2.05	12.05	7.77	4.34	7.60	7.25
250 to 399 beds	9.68	5.49	4.03	9.97	6.71	4.56	15.02	10.57	5.75	9.57	6.80
Teaching Hospitals	7.00	2.85	(0.81)	8.45	4.16	0.07	9.36	6.30	1.87	4.95	4.82
Major	4.82	2.01	(1.15)	7.50	3.12	(0.53)	8.23	4.36	1.87	3.82	4.26
Minor	7.95	3.59	(0.43)	8.77	4.64	0.27	9.94	5.70	1.86	5.33	5.21
Non-Teaching	7.54	3.28	(1.12)	8.34	4.09	(0.05)	9.79	5.34	1.23	5.11	5.19
S&P Bond Rating											
AA(+/-)	10.70	6.77	2.38	12.73	9.69	4.90	13.35	9.70	7.38	9.07	8.79
A+	9.19	6.60	2.75	11.83	8.40	5.07	12.73	9.65	5.77	9.73	9.72
A	8.17	4.51	2.48	10.72	6.55	3.71	10.36	7.43	4.50	6.70	7.33
A-	5.88	3.81	1.30	8.95	5.37	2.57	12.21	7.52	5.28	5.64	5.78
BBB+ and lower	5.67	2.13	(1.22)	5.98	2.91	0.00	8.58	4.44	1.98	4.69	4.08
High Managed Care	7.40	3.69	(0.68)	8.63	4.89	0.76	9.93	6.11	2.41	5.76	5.64
Medium Managed Care	7.46	3.09	(1.01)	8.26	4.00	0.00	9.58	5.28	1.39	4.97	4.94
Low Managed Care	6.84	2.66	(2.20)	8.44	3.08	(2.29)	8.94	3.89	(1.14)	4.64	4.54
Rural Referral Centers	9.80	5.88	2.61	10.74	6.72	3.18	12.55	8.69	5.15	7.99	7.11
Sole Community Providers	7.77	3.75	0.14	8.74	4.48	0.93	10.60	5.84	1.86	5.46	5.91
Disproportionate Share	6.84	2.67	(1.18)	8.18	3.75	(0.05)	9.19	4.81	1.23	4.23	4.34
High Profitability	14.91	10.84	8.94	15.08	10.83	7.50	15.10	11.13	7.30	10.37	8.95
Low Profitability	(2.36)	(4.33)	(8.16)	1.09	(2.14)	(6.07)	3.92	1.05	(2.83)	1.87	2.44

Source: "The Comparative Performance of U.S. Hospitals: 2004 Sourcebook," © 2004, Solucient, LLC. Reprinted with permission.

However, we can "common size" cash by comparing it to total assets. If our cash of $10,000 is one tenth of our total assets and their cash of $5,000 is one tenth of their total assets, then relative to asset size, both organizations are keeping a like amount of cash. This is much more informative. Therefore, the first step in ratio analysis is to create a set of common size ratios. Usually common size ratios are converted to percentages. Thus, rather than referring to cash as being one tenth of total assets, we would refer to it as being 10% of total assets.

To find our common size ratios, we need a key number for comparison. On the balance sheet, the key number is total assets or total equities (i.e., liabilities plus net assets). We calculate the ratio of each asset on the balance sheet as compared to total assets. We calculate the ratio of each liability and net asset account as compared to the total liabilities and net assets. For the statement of operations, all numbers are compared to total revenue. Once we have calculated the common size ratios, we can use them to compare our organization to itself over time, to specific competitors, and to industry-wide statistics.

The common size ratios for CH's balance sheet and statement of operations are presented in Tables 13-1 and 13-3.

The Balance Sheet: Assets

Looking at the balance sheet (see Table 13-1), we can begin to get a general feeling about CH by comparing the common size ratios for 2 years. Note that there is typically some rounding errors in ratio analysis. We could eliminate them by being more precise. For example, in 2007 the ratio of cash to total assets really is 2.6756%. We generally don't bother with such precision. Ratios can't give their users a precise picture of the organiza-

tion. They are meant to serve as general conveyors of broad information. Our concern is if a number is particularly out of line—either unusually high or low. It is virtually impossible to interpret minor changes.

For CH, current assets have remained relatively stable, falling from 31.7% to 31.4% of total assets. Note, however, that accounts receivable have fallen while inventory has risen. Is this good or bad? If accounts receivable have fallen because we are seeing fewer patients or because there are more bad debts, and inventory has risen because CH has not adjusted their purchasing patterns to match the lower patient numbers, then this is bad. It implies that we are accumulating inventory we can't use and are failing to generate revenues from providing patient care. On the other hand, if accounts receivable are down because the organization has been successful in its efforts to collect more promptly and inventory is up because it is needed to support growing patient numbers, then this is a good sign.

Clearly, ratios can't be interpreted in a vacuum. The ratio merely points out what needs to be investigated. The ratio doesn't provide answers in and of itself. In the case of CH, the statement of operations (Table 13-3) shows us that revenue did indeed rise during the fiscal year ending June 30, 2007. It would appear that the changes in accounts receivable and inventory represent a favorable trend.

It is interesting to note that not only is CH increasing its total revenue over time, it appears to be increasing its reliance on premium revenue and other sources of revenue. Both of these categories are increasing in real dollar amounts as well as their respective proportions of total revenue. Once again, there is no easy answer to whether or not this is good or bad. If the premium revenue represents some form of

Table 13-3

Community Hospital
Statement of Operations
For the Years Ended December 31, 2007 and December 31, 2006 (in 000's)

	2007		2006	
Revenues				
Net Patient Services Revenue	$ 180,000	80.4%	$ 159,000	83.2%
Premium Revenue	29,000	12.9%	20,000	10.5%
Other Operating Revenue	15,000	6.7%	12,000	6.3%
Total Revenues From Operations	$ 224,000	100.0%	$ 191,000	100.0%
Expenses				
Salaries and Benefits	$ 75,000	33.5%	$ 68,000	35.6%
Medical Supplies and Drugs	95,000	42.4%	87,000	45.5%
Insurance	15,000	6.7%	12,000	6.3%
Depreciation	20,000	8.9%	16,000	8.4%
Interest	2,000	0.9%	3,000	1.6%
Provision for Bad Debts	5,000	2.2%	3,000	1.6%
Total Expenses From Operations	$ 212,000	94.6%	$ 189,000	99.0%
Excess of Revenues Over Expenses	$ 12,000	5.4%	$ 2,000	1.0%
Unrestricted Contributions	56,000	25.0%	40,000	20.9%
Transfers to Parent	(40,000)	-17.9%	(35,000)	-18.3%
Increase/(Decrease) in Unrestricted Net Assets	$ 28,000	12.5%	$ 7,000	3.7%

managed care carve-out, CH may be increasing its risk with respect to growing expenses to care for patients covered under the carve-out. There may, however, be a specific and well-thought-out plan on the part of management to diversify its revenue sources, and these changes simply make it clear that CH is achieving its goals. As mentioned, ratios are a guide, not an answer. Often they just help us to understand the questions that we need to ask to learn about the financial health of the organization.

Fixed assets (Table 13-1) for CH have increased, not only in absolute terms, but also as a percentage of total assets. After accounting for depreciation that has accumulated on buildings and equipment over their lifetime, we see a rise in net buildings and equipment from 32.4% to 36.8% of total assets.

The Balance Sheet: Liabilities and Net Assets

The current liability common size ratios have remained fairly constant over time (see Table 13-1). Each has risen slightly, which might well have been anticipated given the rise in revenue and inventory noted. As our operations grow and become more profitable, we might expect some growth in current liabilities to match the increases in inventory. In any case, the changes here appear to be modest.

Long-term liabilities (see Table 13-1) have fallen as a percentage of total equities. This is primarily because the organization has not needed to raise funds from the debt market to finance its fixed asset growth. The only caveat is the growth in "Other" long-term debt from $70 to $78 million almost completely offsets the decline in the mortgage payable. In all likelihood, the notes to

the financial statements help to explain this category and its growth.

The common size ratio for total net assets (see Table 13-1) has risen from 19.4% for 2006 to 22.7% for 2007. This is not surprising considering the absolute growth in the excess of revenue over expenses (see Table 13-3). It is also important to note the shift that has taken place within net assets. The growth in net assets is limited to the unrestricted category. Unrestricted net assets have increased from 6.8% in 2006 to 11.0% in 2007. Temporarily and permanently restricted net assets have fallen as a percentage of the total owing to the fact that they have remained constant in dollar terms. Is this good or bad? Ask any finance officer and they will indicate that whereas growth in unrestricted net assets is desirable, the lack of growth in the other two categories may be a problem. It is indicative of a failure on the part of development activities (fundraising). There were no donations to increase endowment in 2007 (permanently restricted net assets), nor even any increases in donations earmarked for specific projects.

Excel Template

Template 11 may be used to calculate common size ratios for your organization's balance sheet. The template is on the Web at www.jbpub.com.

The Statement of Operations

For the statement of operations (Table 13-3), total revenue is the key figure around which all common size ratios are calculated. This year total expenses have fallen in relation to revenue. Assuming that quality has been maintained, this is a favorable trend. By keeping expenses down relative to revenue, surpluses should rise. If we look closer at the changes within expenses for CH, we can see that both salaries and supplies fell as a proportion of total revenues. It would appear this is where CH has gained some efficiency. Although this looks good, internal management should, nevertheless, be very interested in determining why this occurred. If the causes were related to improved efficiency, we want to know that so we can reward the individuals responsible and maintain a higher level of efficiency. On the other hand, if the apparent improvement was due to increased turnover and staff vacancies, the long-run impact may be to hurt our reputation and potentially reduce our surpluses or profits in the longer term.

Therefore, even favorable trends such as reduced expenses should be viewed with caution. Investigation is needed to determine why that change occurred.

For CH, other operating expenses have remained fairly stable, increasing in relative proportion to the dollar increase in total revenue. The excess revenues over expenses, sometimes called the *operating profit*, have increased from 1.0% in 2006 to 5.4% in 2007. This increase is due to the fact that total revenues increased at a faster rate than total expenses.

There are two other changes worthy of note for CH. First, the increase in unrestricted donations from 20.9% of total revenues in 2006 to 25.0% in 2007. This is a rather large increase that in turn helps to increase the overall change in unrestricted net assets at the bottom of the statement. Second, the transfer to parent has actually fallen from 2006 to 2007. Although CH has transferred more dollars in absolute terms ($40 million compared to $35 million the year before), this year's transfer was only 17.9% of total revenue compared to a last year's transfer that was 18.3% of total revenue.

> **Excel Template**
>
> Template 12 may be used to calculate common size ratios for your organization's income statement. The template is on the Web at www.jbpub.com.

Common Size Ratios: Additional Notes

The common size ratios give a starting point. You can quickly get a feel for any unusual changes that have occurred, adjusted for the overall size of assets and the relative amount of revenue. Comparison with specific and industry-wide competition would point out other similarities and differences. For example, our organization has 31.4% of its assets in the current category (see Table 13-1). Is that greater or less than the industry average? If it's substantially greater or less, then you might want to investigate why. Are we in a peculiarly different situation relative to other organizations in our industry?

As mentioned, the key to interpretation of ratios is benchmarks. Without a basis for comparison, it is impossible to reasonably interpret the meaning of a ratio.

LIQUIDITY RATIOS

Liquidity ratios attempt to assess whether an organization is maintaining an appropriate level of liquidity. Too little liquidity raises the possibility of default and bankruptcy. Too much liquidity implies that long-term investments with greater profitability have been missed. Financial officers have to walk a tightrope to maintain enough, but not too much, liquidity.

The most common of the liquidity ratios is the current ratio (Table 13-4), discussed previously. This ratio compares all of the organization's current assets to all of its current liabilities. A common rule of thumb is that the current ratio should be 2.

A second liquidity ratio exists that places even more emphasis on the organization's short-term viability—its ability to continue operations. This ratio is called the *quick ratio*. It compares current assets quickly convertible into cash to current liabilities (see Table 13-4). The concept here is that although not all current assets become cash in the very near term, most current liabilities have to be paid in the very near term. For example, prepaid rent is a current asset, but it is unlikely that we could cash in that prepayment to use to pay our debts. Inventory, although salable, takes time to sell.

The quick ratio compares the organization's cash plus marketable securities plus accounts receivable to its current liabilities. Accounts receivable are considered to be "quick" assets because there are factoring firms that specialize in lending money on receivables or actually buying them outright, so they can be used to generate cash almost immediately. For CH, the quick ratio fell from 1.2 in 2006 to .9 in 2007.

The third liquidity ratio is the *days cash on hand*. Although this ratio looks more complicated than the first two, conceptually it is relatively simple. The numerator of the ratio (cash + marketable securities) is a representation of how much cash or cash equivalents the organization has on hand. The denominator can be best understood by breaking it down into its elements. First, operating expenses less bad debts and depreciation is a representation of the cash operating costs for the year. Bad debts and depreciation are non-cash expenses, so we subtract them out of the annual expenses to get closer to the cash operating costs. Now that we have the cash operating costs for the year we divide by 365 to get a daily operating cost. In other words, the denominator is an estimate of the daily operating cash costs for the organization. When the cash on hand (numerator) is divided by daily operating cash costs (denominator) we have an estimate of the number of days the organization could continue to operate without any additional cash inflows.

For CH, the days cash on hand increased from 69 days in 2006 to 78 days in 2007. Once again, although increasing the number of days cash on hand may be a good thing, too high a value may be an indicator that CH is not using its cash wisely and missing potential returns and investment opportunities.

All of the liquidity ratios have commonly been used as measures of the organization's risk—how likely it is to get into financial difficulty. However, you should be extremely cautious in using these ratios. Three ratios alone do not tell the entire story of an organization. They should be used like clues or

---

Table 13-4 Liquidity Ratios

$$\text{Current Ratio} = \frac{\text{Current Assets}}{\text{Current Liabilities}}$$

$$\text{Quick Ratio} = \frac{\text{Cash + Marketable Securities + Receivables}}{\text{Current Liabilities}}$$

$$\text{Days Cash on Hand} = \frac{\text{Cash + Marketable Securities}}{(\text{Operating Expenses} - \text{Bad Debts} - \text{Depreciation}) / 365}$$

pieces of evidence for the financial analyst who is really acting as a detective. Any one clue can point in the wrong direction.

For example, suppose a hospital has large balances in cash and marketable securities, and its current ratio is 4 or 5. Is this an extremely safe organization? The current ratio by itself leads us to believe that the hospital is very safe. However, what if the hospital is losing money at a rapid rate, and the only thing that staved off bankruptcy was the sale of a major physical asset or investment? The sale generated enough cash to meet immediate needs and left an excess, resulting in the high current and quick ratios. How long will this excess last? If the cash and securities are large relative to current liabilities, but small relative to operating costs or long-term liabilities, then the hospital may still be extremely risky. In this scenario, the days cash on hand may provide better information about the true relationship between cash and the high operating costs.

On the other hand, a very profitable hospital may be in the process of substantially expanding its physical facilities. Because of cash payments related to the expansion, perhaps the current ratio falls to 1.5 and the quick ratio to .6 at year end. Those ratios seem to imply financial weakness. However, within a month or two after the year end, the hospital may be expecting to receive cash from operating its profitable operating activities or perhaps it has already arranged to borrow money for the expansion. This hospital is probably stable. The point is that all of the ratios, when taken together, can supplement the financial statements and the notes to the financial statements. They can point out areas for specific additional investigation. However, no one or two ratios by themselves can, in any way, replace the information in the financial statements, the notes to the financial statements, and other information possessed by management.

Excel Template

Template 13 may be used to calculate liquidity ratios for your organization. The template is on the Web at www.jbpub.com.

EFFICIENCY RATIOS

Whether health care organizations want to maximize their profit/surplus or the quantity and quality of services provided, the organization must operate efficiently. A number of ratios exist that can help an organization to assess how efficiently it is operating and allow for comparison between organizations and over time. These ratios are sometimes referred to as *activity ratios*. The principal *efficiency* or *activity ratios* measure the efficient handling of receivables, payables, and total assets.

Receivables Ratios

One problem faced by most health care organizations is the timely collection of receivables. Once receivables are collected, the money received can be used to pay off loans or it can be invested. This means that once money is received, either we would be paying less interest or we would be earning more interest. Therefore, we want to collect our receivables promptly.

We often think of receivables in terms of how long it takes from billing to collection. A useful aid in analysis is to convert our receivables and our patient revenue into a measure that represents the number of days in accounts receivable (Table 13-5). *Days in accounts receivable* is an easy ratio to calculate and understand once you break it down to its component parts. The numerator—net accounts receivable—is used as a proxy for the amount of money that our patients and their insurers owe us at any point in time, which we ultimately expect to collect. It is important to note that because this figure comes from the balance sheet it technically is the value of accounts receivable on a specific day. We are therefore assuming that the last day of the fiscal year is a good representation of accounts receivable on any given day. If this is not a valid assumption, we can also calculate the average accounts receivable balance by taking the beginning of the year value plus the ending receivables value and dividing by two. This yields the "average" accounts receivable. Alternatively, we can find the average value of receivables at the end of each of the 12 months of the year.

The denominator in the days in accounts receivable ratio is simply the annual patient revenue divided by 365 to yield the average patient revenue per day. Average receivables divided by the average revenue per day yields the number of days the average bill stays a receivable. For CH, the days in accounts receivables is 72 (44,000,000/[224,000,000/365]).

In other words, it is taking CH 72 days to convert a bill into a cash collection. At first thought, you would think that we would want to have this ratio be as low as possible. However, much like the current ratio, we want the days in accounts receivables ratio to be neither too high nor too low. We are really striving for a middle ground, rather than far to one extreme as possible. This is because of the fact that if we try to keep the days in accounts receivables extremely low, our credit manager may attempt to deny credit to anyone that typically pays slowly. This is not necessarily in the best interest of the organization. The services (that the credit manager is denying) may create enough revenue that we benefit even if the customer or insurer is slow to pay.

We therefore want to not only calculate the days in accounts receivables, but we also need to investigate that ratio to see if a short average days in accounts receivables indicates too restrictive a credit policy or if a long days in accounts receivables indicates too loose a credit policy or a lack of sufficient efforts to collect in a timely manner.

One final caution with respect to days in accounts receivable: many health care organizations are dominated by one or two payers such as Medicare or Medicaid. Long-term care facilities, for example, may have as much as 90% of their revenue coming from a state Medicaid program. Programs like Medicaid have been known to skip payments to providers if the annual budget for their state is not passed on a timely basis. The providers typically have no recourse

Table 13-5 Efficiency Ratios

$$\text{Days in Accounts Receivable} = \frac{\text{Net Accounts Receivable}}{\text{(Net Patient Revenue)} / 365}$$

$$\text{Days in Accounts Payable} = \frac{\text{Accounts Payable}}{\text{(Operating Expenses} - \text{Depreciation)} / 365}$$

$$\text{Average Payment Period} = \frac{\text{Current Liabilities}}{\text{(Operating Expenses} - \text{Depreciation)} / 365}$$

$$\text{Total Asset Turnover} = \frac{\text{Total Revenue}}{\text{Total Assets}}$$

and the state ultimately catches up. But, at the time of the skipped payment, the days in accounts receivable rises dramatically (the organization is carrying twice the normal receivables). Once again, this points to the fact that all ratios need to be taken with a grain of salt and the analyst must look at the context within which the specific numerical value exists. It also shows the importance of ratios such as days cash on hand. Can the organization sustain a period without cash collections?

Payables Ratios

The same type of ratio calculated for receivables can be calculated with respect to payables (Table 13-5). The *days in accounts payable ratio* gives us a measure of how many days it takes our organization to pay its bills. Like the receivables ratio, a middle position is desired. Pay your bills too quickly and you forgo the opportunity to earn more interest on your cash. Take too long to pay your bills and you run the risk of payment penalties (additional costs) or being denied credit by your suppliers in the future.

The calculation of days in accounts payable takes the same form as the receivables ratio. The numerator is the accounts payable balance from the balance sheet. The denominator is an estimate of the daily operating costs. This estimate is obtained by taking the annual operating expenses, less depreciation, and dividing by 365. When combined, the numerator and denominator yield the number of days it takes our organization to pay its bills.

For CH, the days in accounts payable was 110 days in 2007 up from 105 days in 2006. These values are above what most health care organizations run, and the fact that it is increasing is not a good sign.

An additional measure of an organization's payment pattern is the *average payment period ratio.* This ratio is similar to the days in accounts receivables described above, but includes all current liabilities in the numerator. By including all current liabilities, this ratio is a broader measure of an organization's payment record. Average payment period incorporates the fact that there are short-term creditors not included in accounts payable. In the case of CH, their average payment period was 179 days! One doesn't need an advanced degree in finance to know that this is higher than what most organizations want.

CH would have to take a very close look at why it appears to be taking so long to pay its bills. They may be making their cash position look favorable by holding on to cash too long and not paying bills. This could ultimately threaten their ability to get supplies in a timely manner. On the other hand, this ratio may be artificially inflated by inclusion of items such as deferred revenues. *Deferred revenues* represent amounts that customers (such as health maintenance organizations) have prepaid for care. Until we provide patient care, we show the amount as a liability. Once we provide care, we eliminate the liability from our balance sheet and record revenue. Because we never really intend to repay these advances (we intend to provide care), it is not as critical if these amounts remain on the balance sheet for a number of days.

Total Asset Turnover

A final efficiency ratio is the *total asset turnover ratio.* This ratio compares total operating revenue to total assets. The more revenues an organization can generate per dollar of assets, the more efficient it is, other things being equal. If we divide 2007 revenue of $224 million (from Table 13-3) by total assets of $598 million (from Table 13-1), the ratio of 0.37 indicates that CH generates $0.37 of revenue for every $1 in assets. Relative to most health care organizations that generate approximately $1 of revenue for every $1 invested in assets, this is very low. This is another piece of the financial puzzle that CH would need to investigate to determine the cause and to see if there are ways to use their assets more efficiently and thereby generate additional revenue.

Excel Template

Template 14 may be used to calculate efficiency ratios for your organization. The template is on the Web at www.jbpub.com.

SOLVENCY RATIOS

One of the primary focuses on the organization's riskiness occurs through examination of its solvency ratios. Unlike the liquidity ratios that are concerned with the organization's ability to meet its obligations in the very near future, solvency ratios take more of a long-term view. They attempt to determine if the organization has overextended itself through the use of financial leverage. That is, does the organization have principal and interest payment obligations exceeding its ability to pay, not only now, but into the future as well? These ratios are sometimes referred to as *leverage* or *capital structure ratios*.

Three of the most common of the solvency ratios are the *interest coverage ratio* (also referred to as the times interest earned ratio), the *debt service coverage ratio*, and the *debt to net assets ratio* or debt to equity ratio in for-profit organizations (Table 13-6). The interest and debt service coverage ratios focus on the ability to meet interest and principal payments arising from liabilities. The debt to net assets ratio focuses on the protective cushion that net assets (or owner's equity) provides for creditors. If a bankruptcy does occur, creditors can share in the organization's assets before the owners can claim any of their equity. The more equity (or net assets) that the organization has, the greater likelihood that the organization's assets will be great enough to protect the claims of all the creditors.

The interest coverage ratio compares funds available to pay interest to the total amount of interest that has to be paid. The funds available for interest are the organization's profits (excess of revenues over expenses) before paying interest (in for-profit organizations, you would also want to add back in taxes that were paid). As long as the profit before interest is greater than the amount of interest, the organization will have enough money to pay the interest owed. Therefore, excess of revenue over expenses plus interest is divided by interest expense to calculate this ratio. The higher this ratio is, the more comfortable creditors feel.

Table 13-6 Solvency Ratios

$$\text{Interest Coverage} = \frac{\text{Excess of Revenues Over Expenses} + \text{Interest Expense}}{\text{Interest Expense}}$$

$$\text{Debt Service Coverage} = \frac{\text{Excess of Revenues Over Expenses} + \text{Interest Expense} + \text{Depreciation Expense}}{\text{Interest} + \text{Principal Payments}}$$

$$\frac{\text{Long-Term}}{\text{Debt to Net Assets}} = \frac{\text{Long-Term Debt}}{\text{Net Assets}}$$

For CH in 2007, the excess of revenues over expenses was $12 million with $2 million in interest expense (Table 13-3). The interest coverage ratio therefore is 7.0, or (12 + 2)/2. This is a significant improvement from 2006, when the excess of revenues over expenses was $2 million and the interest was $3 million. In that year, the interest coverage was 1.7.

However, we should be careful in our use of the term *improvement*. From a creditor's point of view, this is an improvement because profits are up relative to interest, creating a greater cushion of safety. From the organization's point of view, whether this is an improvement or not depends on its attitude toward risk and profits. For example, if the organization doesn't mind risk, it could have provided more charity care, increasing expenses and lowering profits. The interest coverage ratio would be lower, but more free care would have been provided.

The debt service coverage ratio builds on the interest coverage ratio and provides a broader and more comprehensive look at the organization's ability to pay its long-term debt. In the case of the debt service coverage ratio, the numerator is the same as in the interest coverage ratio but we add the depreciation expense so that we get an approximation for the available cash flow. The denominator is then both the interest and the principal payments.

In the case of CH we get a debt service coverage ratio of 2.8 for 2007. To calculate this ratio, we need to pull information from both the statement of operations and the statement of cash flows. The excess of revenues over expenses of $12 million along with the interest expense of $2 million and the depreciation expense of $20 million comes from the statement of operations (Table 13-3). The principal payment of $10 million comes from the statement of cash flows (Table 11-5).

The final solvency ratio is the *long-term debt to net assets ratio*. This ratio measures the proportion of debt to net assets and gives a good sense of the overall debt burden the organization has. In the case of CH, the long-term debt to net assets ratio is 2.7. This means that there is $2.70 of long-term debt for every $1 in net assets. CH would certainly be considered highly leveraged. On the positive side, the debt to net assets ratio has improved for CH from 3.4 in 2006.

Excel Template

Template 15 may be used to calculate solvency ratios for your organizations. The template is included on the Web at www.jbpub.com.

PROFITABILITY RATIOS

When all is said and done, the key focus of accounting and finance tends to be on profits. Profitability ratios attempt to show how well the organization did, given the level of risk and types of risk it actually assumed during the year.

If we compare net income to that of the competition, it is an inadequate measure. Suppose that the chief competitor of CH had earnings of $57 million this year, and CH made only $19 million. Did the competitor have a better year? Not necessarily. It earned three times as much money, but perhaps it required four times as much in resources to do it. Therefore, a number of profitability ratios exist to help in evaluating the organization's performance.

Margin Ratios

Margin ratios are one common class of profitability ratios. Health care organizations commonly compute their total margin and their operating margin as a percentage of revenues. These ratios (Table 13-7) are nothing more than common size ratios we calculated previously. For CH in 2007, the total margin was 10% (total increase in net assets $28 million divided by total revenue of $280 million, which is the combination of operating revenue and nonoperating revenue). The operating margin for CH in 2007 was 5.4% ($12 million divided by $224 million). These margins are often watched closely, as changes can be early warning signals of serious problems.

RETURN ON INVESTMENT (ROI) RATIOS

Another broad category of profitability measures falls under the heading of return on investment (ROI). There are many definitions for ROI, although individual organizations usually select one definition and use that as a measure of both individual and organization performance. Because we cannot know the specific definition an organization has chosen, we discuss a variety of ROI measures in this section. Even if none of the ones discussed here is exactly the same as that chosen by your organization, you should gain enough from the discussion to understand the strengths and weaknesses of whatever ROI measure(s) your organization uses.

Return on assets (ROA) is an ROI measure that evaluates the organization's return or net income relative to the asset base used to generate the income. If we could invest $100 in each of two different investments, and one generated twice as much income as the other, we would prefer the investment generating twice as much income (assuming the levels of risk had been the same).

Therefore, the organization that generates more income, relative to the amount of investment, is doing a better job, other things equal. If we divide the profit earned by the amount of assets employed to generate that profit, we get the ROA. A high ROA is better than a small one. The ROA measure is particularly good for evaluating division managers. It focuses on how well they used the assets entrusted to them.

Return on net assets (RONA) is another measure of profitability that allows the analyst to focus on how well the organization did in earning a RONA (see Table 13-7). In the case of CH, the 2007 ROA was 2% ($12 million excess of revenue over expenses divided by $598 million in assets) and the RONA was 9% ($12 million excess of revenue over expenses divided by $136 million in net assets).

Table 13-7 Profitability Ratios

$$\text{Total Margin} = \frac{\text{Total Net Income or Total Increase in Net Assets}}{\text{Total Revenue}}$$

$$\text{Operating Margin} = \frac{\text{Excess of Revenue Over Expenses}}{\text{Operating Revenue}}$$

$$\text{Return on Assets} = \frac{\text{Excess of Revenues Over Expenses}}{\text{Total Assets}}$$

$$\text{Return on Net Assets} = \frac{\text{Excess of Revenues Over Expenses}}{\text{Net Assets}}$$

Although ROA is good for evaluating managers but inadequate for evaluating the overall organization, RONA is good for evaluating overall organization performance but not for manager evaluation. Except for very top officers of the organization, managers do not control whether the organization borrows money to maintain or expand operations. Most managers are simply trying to use the funds that the finance officers have provided them most efficiently. If two managers operated their organizations exactly the same, except that one was financed substantially with debt and the other was financed almost exclusively with donations, the organizations would have substantially different RONAs for two reasons. First, the net assets are different for the two organizations; because one organization had more donations than the other, the denominator of the ratio will be different. Second, the interest expense differs because one organization borrowed less than the other, so the excess of revenues over expenses are not the same. Therefore, the numerator of the ratio is different. How can we evaluate what part of the organization's results was caused by reasons other than the leverage decision, and what part was caused by the specific decision regarding financial leverage?

So, the manager who makes a decision to borrow rather than to go the more difficult route of raising donations may be held accountable on a RONA basis. But if the Board makes the decision to not bother with a fundraising campaign and instructs the manager to borrow money, then the manager should not be held accountable for the impact of that decision.

RONA is a useful measure of the income that the organization was able to generate relative to the amount of net assets and contributions in the organization. RONA includes the effect caused by the organization's degree of leverage (i.e., how much it borrowed). To remove the impact of leverage from our evaluation, we should use ROA. This eliminates the problem with respect to the denominator of the RONA ratio. The asset base or denominator of the ROA ratio is the same whether the source of the money used to acquire the assets is debt or equity. However, ROA leaves a problem with the numerator. The return, or numerator (the net income), is affected by the amount of interest the organization pays. For this reason, the measure of ROA often used for evaluation abstracting from the leverage decision is calculated using something called *delevered net income.*

Delevered net income means recalculating the organization's income by assuming that it had no interest expense at all. In doing this, we can put organizations with different decisions regarding the use of borrowed money all on a comparable basis. We can see how profitable each organization was relative to the assets it used regardless of their source. We have completely separated any profitability (or loss) created by having used borrowed money instead of contributed capital. The way we delever net income is to take the organization's operating margin (income before interest and taxes) and calculate taxes directly on that amount, ignoring interest. The result is a net income based on the assumption that there was no interest expense.

This should not lead the reader to believe that all organizations calculate ROA in exactly the same way. Some organizations use assets net of depreciation as the basis for comparison. This is how the assets appear on the balance sheet. Some organizations ignore depreciation and use gross assets as a base. The reason for this is to avoid causing an organization or division to appear to have a very high return on assets simply because its assets are very old and fully depreciated.

Such fully depreciated assets cause the base of the ratio to be very low and, therefore, the resulting ratio to be very large. Along the same lines, some organizations use replacement cost instead of historical cost to place divisions in an equal position.

Despite any of these adjustments, use of any of the ROA measures for evaluation of managers creates undesired incentives. Suppose the organization is happy to accept any project with an after-tax rate of return of 20%. One division of the organization currently has an ROA of 30%, and a proposed project that would have a 25% ROA is being evaluated. The manager of the division wants to reject the project entirely if he or she is evaluated based on ROA. The 25% project, even though profitable, and perhaps better than anything else the organization could do with their money, will bring down that division's weighted average ROA, which is currently 30%. Even though the project is good for the organization, it would hurt the manager's performance evaluation.

For this reason we recommend an ROI concept called *residual income* (RI). Under this approach, the organization specifies a minimum required ROA rate, using one of the various approaches discussed. For each project being evaluated, we multiply the amount of asset investment required for the project by the required ROA rate. The result is subtracted from the profits anticipated from the project. If the project is expected to earn more than the proposed investment multiplied by the required rate, then there will be a residual left over after the subtraction. A division manager would be evaluated on the residual left over from all his or her projects combined.

For example, suppose that 20% was considered to be an acceptable rate to the organization. Currently all projects for the division earn 30%. Suppose further that a project requiring an investment of $100,000 of assets was proposed. If this new project would earn a profit of $25,000, or 25% ROA, it would be rejected by a manager evaluated on an ROA basis. From an ROA basis, the 25% would lower the currently achieved 30% average. For RI, we would multiply the $100,000 investment by the 20% ROA required rate, getting a result of $20,000. When the $20,000 is subtracted from the profit of $25,000, there is a $5,000 RI. The manager is considered to have increased his or her RI by $5,000.

The advantage of this method is that if the organization would like to undertake any project earning a return of more than 20%, division managers will have an incentive to accept all such projects. This is because all projects earning more than 20% will cover the minimum desired 20% ROA and have some excess left over. This excess adds to the manager's total RI. Thus, RI motivates the manager to do what is also in the best interests of the organization.

The reader can readily see that ROI is not a simple topic. The finance officers of most organizations spend a fair amount of time considering the implications of various forms of ROI for both motivation and evaluation. Unfortunately, many organizations use just one ROI measure for the organization and its managers. In attempting to make the measure serve multiple roles, the ROI measures used often are so complex that they are difficult to understand. The net result often is that ROI measures do not motivate the way they are intended to and do not provide fair measures of performance.

Excel Template

Template 16 may be used to calculate profitability ratios for your organization. The template is included on the Web at www.jbpub.com.

KEY CONCEPTS

Ratio—Any number compared to another number. Ratios are calculated by dividing one number into another.

Benchmarks—An organization's ratios can be compared to ratios for the same organization from prior years and to ratios of a specific competitor and to ratios for the entire industry.

Common size ratios—All numbers on the balance sheet are compared to total assets or total liabilities plus net assets, and all numbers on the income statement are compared to total revenue. This makes interorganization or interperiod comparison of specific numbers such as cash more meaningful.

Liquidity ratios—Assess the organization's ability to meet its current obligations as they become due.

Efficiency ratios—Assess the efficiency with which the organization manages its resources, such as inventory and receivables.

Solvency ratios—Assess the organization's ability to meet its interest payments and long-term obligations as they become due.

Profitability ratios—Assess how profitable the organization was and how well it was managed by comparing profits to the amount of resources invested in the organization and used to generate the profits earned.

TEST YOUR KNOWLEDGE

See www.jbpub.com/catalog/0763726753/supplements.htm.

CHAPTER 14

Working Capital Management and Banking Relationships

WORKING CAPITAL MANAGEMENT

An organization's *net working capital,* or working capital, is its current assets less its current liabilities. This chapter focuses on *working capital management:* techniques and approaches designed to maximize the benefit of short-term resources and minimize the cost of short-term obligations.

Working capital is based on a cycle of outflows and inflows. For example, Keepuwell Clinic might use cash to buy supplies. The supplies are used to treat patients. The employees providing the health care must also be paid. When the patient is treated and a service is delivered, the clinic can bill the patient or insurer and thereby create a receivable. Once those receivables are collected, the cycle starts over and that money can be used to buy more supplies and pay workers to treat more patients.

The cycle may be delicately balanced. At the beginning of the cycle, Keepuwell Clinic may have just enough to pay for supplies and wages if it received payments promptly from its patients. If Keepuwell issues bills once a month instead of weekly or daily, it may be more convenient for the bookkeeper, but it postpones the collection of cash. That cash is needed as soon as possible so that Keepuwell can cover its expenses.

In performing working capital management, it is the role of the manager to ensure that there is adequate cash on hand to meet the organization's needs and also to minimize the cost of that cash. To do this, the manager must carefully monitor and control cash inflows and outflows. Cash not immediately needed should be invested, earning a return for the organization. An organization should not keep excess inventory. The money spent to pay for inventory that is not yet needed could be better used by the organization for some other purpose. At a minimum, the money could be earning interest. Similarly, if the organization pays its bills before they are due, it also loses interest it could have earned if it had left the cash in its savings account for a little longer.

SHORT-TERM RESOURCES

The most essential element of working capital is cash. When accountants refer to *cash* they mean both currency on hand as well as amounts that can be withdrawn from bank accounts. A second type of short-term resource is *marketable securities.* These are investments, such as stock and debt, that can be bought and sold in financial markets, such as the New York Stock Exchange. In most organizations, accounts receivables and inventory are also important parts of working capital. These short-term resources are discussed in this section.

Cash

There are three principal reasons that organizations want to keep some cash on hand or in their bank accounts. First, cash is needed for the normal daily transactions of any activity. For example, cash is needed to pay employees and suppliers. Second, although many activities can be anticipated, managers can never foresee everything that might happen. Experience has shown that it makes sense for organizations to have a safety cushion available for emergencies. A third reason for holding cash is to have it available if an attractive investment opportunity arises.

Given these three reasons to hold cash, one might think that the more cash we have, the better. That is not the case. Cash earns a very low rate of return (e.g., bank savings account interest) at best. If we use our cash to buy buildings and equipment we can probably earn higher profits. But then we wouldn't have cash for transactions and emergencies. At the other extreme, we can keep all our resources in cash, but then we wouldn't earn much of a profit. In practice, managers must find a middle ground, trying to keep enough cash available, but not too much.

Short-Term Cash Investments and Marketable Securities

Cash should be earning a return whenever possible. Organizations should have specific policies that result in cash and checks received being deposited promptly into inter-est-bearing accounts. In fact, even after a check is written to make a payment, it is possible to continue to earn interest on the money. The period from when you write a check until it clears your bank account is called the *float.* Many banks have arrangements that allow money to be automatically transferred from an interest-bearing account to a checking account as checks are received for payment.

Although interest-bearing accounts are better than noninterest-bearing accounts, they pay relatively low rates of interest. There are a variety of alternative short-term investments that have the potential to earn a higher rate of return. In a world of no free lunches, however, there is generally a trade off when one obtains a higher rate of return. The two most common trade offs are decreased liquidity and increased risk. Decreased liquidity means that the money is not immediately accessible. For example, *certificates of deposit* (CDs) pay higher interest rates than savings accounts, but there is often a penalty for early withdrawal.

Although CDs may tie up money for a period of time, they are generally quite safe. Other investments hold promise of even higher rates of return, but entail greater risks. Marketable securities can be sold almost immediately and cash from the sale can be received within a few days. However, such investments are subject to market fluctuations. The prices of stocks and bonds may go up and down significantly, even on a daily basis.

Other Short-Term Investment Options

Other options exist for short-term investments of cash. A *Treasury bill* (often called a *T-bill*) is a debt security issued by the U.S. government. Maturities range from 4 weeks to 1 year. If the bill is held until it matures, the federal government guarantees to pay the maturity value. T-bills can be purchased directly from the federal government without a fee through the Treasury Direct system online at www.publicdebt.treas.gov. It is possible to sell a T-bill prior to its maturity date. Most stock brokerage firms will buy or sell T-bills for a fee of about $50.

Another alternative is money market funds. These investments tend to pay a rate below that of CDs, but competitive with T-bills and higher than the rate paid on a bank savings account. Interest is earned daily and money can be deposited or withdrawn at any time. Although the investment has no guarantee, money market funds are generally considered to be reasonably safe investments and they are very convenient to use.

The next type of money market instrument is a *negotiable certificate of deposit* issued by a U.S. bank. A negotiable CD can be sold to someone else, just as a bond can be sold. Sales commissions are incurred and the value of the CD at the time of sale depends on what has happened to market interest rates and the creditworthiness of the lender during the time since the investment was made.

Another type of money market instrument is *commercial paper*. Commercial paper generally represents a note payable issued by a corporation. Typical maturities are less than 1 year, and the interest rate is higher than a T-bill. The buyer of the paper is lending money to a corporation. There is a risk, albeit small, that the corporation will not repay the loan.

Repurchase agreements, or *repos*, are types of short-term investments that are collateralized by securities. Repos may be for as short a period of time as overnight. The organization with idle cash provides it to the borrower at an agreed-upon interest rate, which may fluctuate daily. Although repos are quite liquid, they do have a variety of risks.

For example, if the borrower defaults, the collateral may turn out to be insufficient to cover the full investment.

Commercial paper, negotiable CDs, and repos would generally be suitable only for organizations that have substantial amounts of cash (perhaps over a million dollars) available for short-term investment. These investments can be quite complicated and should be used only by organizations that employ competent advisors knowledgeable in their intricacies and potential risks.

Accounts Receivable

One should always attempt to collect accounts receivable as quickly as possible. The sooner we collect all of our receivables, the sooner the organization has the cash for its use, at least for investment in an interest-bearing bank account. Also, the longer we allow an account receivable to be outstanding, the lower the chances that it will ever be collected.

As discussed in Chapter 2, the health care reimbursement system is very complex. In most cases, the patient does not simply come in, receive services, and pay the bill. The combination of direct patient payments and third-party insurance payments requires significant management attention. Next, we discuss specific accounts receivables management practices, followed by a broader discussion of how health care managers must manage the entire revenue cycle. This broader revenue cycle management encompasses the entire process from initial patient scheduling to collection of receivables. Accounts receivable are collected as a result of a cycle of activities as depicted in Figure 14-1.

As you can see, there are a number of potential bottlenecks that delay the full conversion of a bill to cash. The faster and more accurately we compile the information

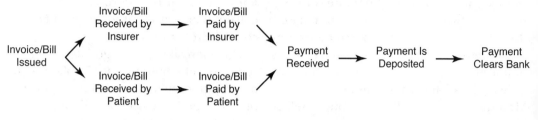

Figure 14-1 The Receivables Cycle

needed to issue an invoice, and the sooner we actually issue the invoice, the faster payment can be expected to be received.

Management of accounts receivable does not stop when we issue an invoice. We need to establish credit policies that reduce the amount of money lost because patients fail to pay the amounts they owe us. We also need to monitor unpaid receivables to minimize such losses. An aging schedule, showing how long our receivables have been outstanding, is a very helpful device. When receivables are collected, there should be specific procedures to safeguard the cash until its ultimate deposit in the bank.

Credit Policies

Credit policies relate to deciding which customers or patients are allowed to make purchases on account. Organizations require some (or all) customers to pay cash at the time of purchase if there is a high risk that payment would not be received later. However, by excluding individuals or organizations from buying goods or services on account, we may lose their business. You want to give credit terms that are as good as the competition, but don't want to give credit to customers or patients who wind up never paying their bills. This requires a skillful credit manager to weigh the risks versus the benefits of extending credit to specific customers.

Of course, it should also be noted that emergency patients must always be provided

with care prior to collecting payment. In fact care must be provided before you even request insurance information. Hospitals with emergency rooms are not allowed to pick and choose their patients. Until it is medically determined that a situation is not an emergency, care must be provided without consideration of whether payment will be collected. On the other hand, once emergency care is provided and the patient is in the system, the health care provider must be sure to go back and collect the information needed for accurate and timely billing.

The Billing Process

The activities concentrated around issuing bills are critical. They must be done quickly, but also correctly. Although this basic point is true for all health care organizations, it is especially true for hospitals. The complexity of the reimbursement system makes both accuracy and timeliness more difficult. In recent years, however, there have been enormous strides made in the automation of data collection (the electronic medical record) and the subsequent patient classification and billing systems deployed by hospitals. Inaccurate data for a hospital stay can often result in a claims denial and ultimately a complete failure to collect any payment for service. Some health care organizations now have systems in place that enable the generation of a bill almost immediately upon discharge. For any one bill, it might not seem to matter if there are a few delays. However, when all bills are considered, the impact of prompt billing is significant.

Electronic Billing and Collections

One method to speed collection is electronic billing. In addition to allowing faster collection, electronic billing may prove to be less expensive to process than paper billing because it uses less labor. Electronic billing also allows for quicker communication of problems.

The vast majority of health care providers process their billing and collections with third-party payers electronically. Although there are many different insurers, there has been a great deal of standardization of claims forms, easing some of the burden on providers. Yet it remains a complex and sometimes slow process.

Direct electronic collections from patients can also be used to help reduce the time be-

tween billing and cash collections. Electronic collections from patients can take many forms such as credit or debit cards at the time of service, credit or debit cards via the phone after billing, or online payments after billing. Clearly, if your organization can draw money directly from patients' bank accounts, it can increase the speed of collections and reduce the amount of bad debts.

Aging of Receivables

Once bills have been issued, it is important for the organization to monitor receivables and to follow up on unpaid bills. A useful tool for this process is an accounts receivable *aging schedule*. An aging schedule shows how long it has been between the current date and the date when uncollected bills were issued. For example, at the end of July, a summary aging schedule for the Keepuwell Clinic might appear as the example in Table 14-1.

Table 14-1	Keepuwell Clinic Receivables Aging Schedule As of December 31, 2007				
PAYER	**1–30 Days**	**31–60 Days**	**61–90 Days**	**>90 Days**	**Total**
By Total Dollars					
Various Insurance Companies	$175,463	$25,674	$14,562	$2,567	$218,266
Keepuwell County School District	115,935	11,327	1,674	273	129,209
Prevention First Insurance Company	31,732	10,378	4,389	1,936	48,435
Individual Patients	22,419	15,478	7,321	3,197	48,415
Total	$345,549	$62,857	$27,946	$7,973	$444,325
By Percentage					
Various Insurance Companies	80.4%	11.8%	6.7%	1.2%	100.0%
Keepuwell County School District	89.7%	8.8%	1.3%	0.2%	100.0%
Prevention First Insurance Company	65.5%	21.4%	9.1%	4.0%	100.0%
Individual Patients	46.3%	32.0%	15.1%	6.6%	100.0%
Total	77.8%	14.1%	6.3%	1.8%	100.0%

In Table 14-1, we notice that the largest share of Keepuwell's receivables is from various insurance companies. Keepuwell also has a couple of large receivables outstanding with the Keepuwell County School District and a specific insurance company (Prevention First). Finally, Keepuwell groups all of the individual patients with outstanding receivables together for this report. We can see from the bottom half of the aging schedule that 78% of Keepuwell's receivables have been outstanding for less than 1 month. Less than 2% of its receivables are outstanding for more than 90 days. In the period shortly after bills are issued, in general individual patients are the slowest to pay, with only 46% collected in the first month. Prevention First Insurance Company also appears to be a slow payer, with only 66% collected in the first month, 9% collected in the 61- to 90-day period, and 4% still outstanding after 90 days.

Excel Template

You may use Template 17 to prepare an aging schedule for your organization. The template is on the Web at www.jbpub.com.

The aging schedule is a valuable tool because problem areas can be quickly identified. Efforts to collect payment should begin as soon as the invoice is issued. If anything goes beyond the current column (i.e., 1 to 30 days), there should be a formal procedure, such as the issuance of a reminder statement. If an account exceeds 60 days, there should be procedures such as mailing another statement, often colored pink to get greater attention. The "over-90-day" category in an aging schedule is a particular concern, even though it may be a small part of the total. Amounts in that category probably reflect problems encountered in processing

the bills or else an inability or unwillingness to pay. All organizations should have specific follow-up procedures for accounts that fall into this category. These procedures should include not only monthly statements, but also late charges and telephone calls to determine why payment has not been made. The longer an invoice goes unpaid, the less likely it will ever be paid.

In some cases, it is necessary to use a collection agency if other efforts have failed. This is a costly approach, since collection agencies retain as much as half of all amounts that they are successful in collecting.

Lockboxes

Some organizations have payments sent directly to a *lockbox* rather than to the organization itself. Lockboxes are usually post office boxes that are emptied by the bank rather than the organization. The bank opens the envelopes with the payments and deposits them directly into the organization's account.

One advantage of this approach is that the bank empties the box and deposits the money at least once a day. This gets the money into interest-bearing accounts faster than if it had to go through the organization. Second, use of a lockbox tends to substantially decrease the risk that receipts will be lost or stolen.

Inventory Management

Careful management of inventory can also save money for the organization. The lower the level of inventory kept on hand, the less you have paid out to suppliers, and the greater the amount of money kept in your own interest-bearing savings accounts. On the other hand, for many organizations, there are uncertainties that require inventory both for current use and as a safety measure. Management must develop systems to ensure adequate availability of inventory when needed while keeping overall levels as low as possible.

Centralized storing of inventory should be used if possible. If separate locations for inventory are created, convenience rises but so do costs. The more separate storage sites, the greater the amount of each inventory item the organization is likely to have. The ordering process should also be as centralized as possible to minimize employee time spent processing orders and maximize the possibility of volume discounts.

Economic Order Quantity

There are a variety of costs related to inventory in addition to the purchase price. We must have physical space to store it, we may need to pay to insure it, and there are costs related to placing an order and having it shipped. A method called the *economic order quantity* (EOQ) considers all of these factors in calculating the optimum amount of inventory to order at one time.

The more inventory ordered at one time, the sooner we pay for inventory (taking money out of our investments or interest-bearing accounts) and the greater the costs for things such as inventory storage. These are called *carrying* or *holding* costs. On the other hand, if we keep relatively little inventory on hand to keep carrying costs low, we will have to order inventory more often. That drives *ordering* costs up. EOQ balances these two factors to find the optimal amount to order at one time.

There are two categories of carrying costs. These are *capital cost* and *out-of-pocket costs*. The *capital cost* is the cost related to having paid for inventory, as opposed to using those resources for other alternative uses. At a minimum this is the foregone interest that could have been earned on the money paid for in-

ventory. *Out-of-pocket costs* are other costs related to holding inventory, including rent on space where inventory is kept, insurance and taxes on the value of inventory, the cost of annual inventory counts, the losses due to obsolescence and date-related expirations, and the costs of damage, loss, and theft.

Ordering costs include the cost of having an employee spend time placing orders, the shipping and handling charges for the orders, and the cost of correcting errors when orders are placed. The more orders, the more errors.

There is an offsetting dynamic in inventory management. The more orders per year, the less inventory that needs to be on hand at any given time, and therefore the lower the carrying cost. However, the more orders per year, the greater the amount the organization spends on placing orders, shipping and handling costs, and error correction. The total costs of inventory are the sum of the amount paid for inventory plus the carrying costs plus the ordering costs.

Total Inventory Cost = Purchase Cost + Carrying Cost + Ordering Cost

The goal of inventory management is to minimize this total without reducing the quality of services the organization provides.

We use N for the total number of units of inventory ordered per year, C for the annual cost to carry one unit of inventory, and O for the costs related to placing one order. The EOQ represents the optimal number of units to order at one time.

Suppose that Keepuwell Clinic pays $20 per box of tongue depressors. They buy 200 boxes per year. Each time they place an order, it takes a paid clerk $5 worth of time to process the order. The delivery cost is $10 per order. Thus, $15 is the total ordering cost. Keepuwell earns an average of 6% interest on invested money. Therefore, the capital part of the carrying cost is $1.20 per box per year (6% × $20 price = $1.20). Other carrying costs (such as storage and insurance) are estimated to be $2.40 per box per year. Therefore the total carrying costs are $3.60 per box per year.

The formula to determine the optimal number to order at one time is:

$$EOQ = \sqrt{\frac{2 \, ON}{C}}$$

where EOQ is the optimal amount to order each time.

$$EOQ = \sqrt{\frac{2 \times \$15 \times 200}{\$3.60}}$$

$$= 41$$

This result indicates that we should order 41 boxes at a time to minimize costs related to acquiring and holding inventory.

Excel Template

Template 18 may be used to calculate the EOQ for your organization. The template is on the Web at www.jbpub.com.

The basic EOQ model as presented here makes a number of assumptions that are often not true. For example, it assumes that any number of units can be purchased. In some cases an item might only be sold in certain quantities, such as hundreds or dozens. Another assumption is that the price per unit does not change if we order differing numbers of units with each order. It is possible that we might get a quantity discount for large orders. Such a discount could offset some of the higher carrying cost related to large orders. Managers should adjust the EOQ based on the impact of these issues.

Another assumption is that we use up our last unit of an item just when the next shipment arrives. A delay in processing, however, could cause inventory to arrive late, and we might run out of certain items. To avoid negative consequences of such stock outs, we might want to keep a safety stock on hand. How large should that safety stock be? That depends on how long it takes to get more inventory if we start to run out, and how critical the consequences of running out are.

Clearly, certain health care providers (like emergency departments) can't afford to run out of certain life-saving inventories. It is useful for organizations to categorize inventory by the potential threat to a patient's life to help determine the need and subsequent size of a safety stock.

Just-in-Time Inventory

One aggressive approach to inventory management is called *just-in-time* (JIT) inventory. This method argues that carrying costs should be driven to an absolute minimum. This is accomplished by having inventory arrive just as it is needed for use. The advantages are obvious: no storage costs, reduced handling costs, minimum breakage, and no need to pay for inventory before you need it. However, there are clear disadvantages as well: increased ordering and shipping costs, and the risk that it will be necessary to stop providing service if inventory doesn't arrive as it is needed.

The application of JIT really centers on how close one can come to the ideal. There are invariably problems when implementing a JIT system. For any organization, workflow does not necessarily proceed in an orderly manner. There are peaks and valleys in demand. Such variability creates major challenges for the implementation of a JIT system.

Once again, the key piece for health care organizations is the risk associated for failing to have a specific piece of inventory on hand when needed. Health care organizations may want to apply JIT concepts and approaches to certain categories of inventory that carry less risk.

MANAGING THE REVENUE CYCLE

We mentioned the concept of revenue cycle management. Today's health care system is so complex, both in the delivery of services as well as the billing and collection of payments, that managers need to be focused on more than just accounts receivables management as reviewed. Managing receivables is only part of the revenue cycle. In fact, for many health care providers, the revenue cycle begins when an appointment is scheduled. Next is a brief description of each of the main steps within the revenue cycle. Each step needs attention and often provides opportunities for improvement and thereby reduction in the revenue cycle and faster cash in the bank.

Scheduling

The registration information collected either at the time of scheduling or after scheduling via a pre-registration mechanism is some of the most critical information the organization needs to guarantee smooth and timely payment after services have been provided. This information includes demographics and insurance information and can set the stage for the rest of the revenue cycle.

Point of Service

The next step in the revenue cycle is often at the time of service when the patient shows up for care. The patient "check-in" and/or "check-out" provides a unique opportunity to collect data that were not collected as part of scheduling or pre-registration. This step also provides the opportunity for direct collection of any patient co-pays and/or balances that greatly reduce/eliminate the receivables.

Coding

As mentioned, the ability to accurately code at the time of service is critical to the timely collection of payment. Coding represents the translation of services provided into billable charges. The requirements for coding may vary by payer; therefore, compliance is critical. A well-organized system of coding is essential in today's health care system. Automated systems help to streamline the process of coding, but ultimately there are many opportunities for human error and delay. In some cases, coding systems are imposed on the provider. Medicare uses diagnosis-related group (DRG) codes for inpatients. Current protocol terminology (CPT) codes are commonly used by many payers for outpatient care. Other coding systems exist as well.

Billing and Claims

The major issues in this step of the revenue cycle were discussed previously. The main issue is the timely filing of claims and subsequent tracking of denials and prompt resolution of problems. Once again, automation, such as electronic filing of claims, can greatly improve the efficiency of this step in the cycle.

Third-Party and Patient Collections

This step in the revenue cycle is really the solid management of receivables. This includes development of aging schedules and follow-up on slow payers. It is also critical at this stage to match insurance and patient payments to make sure that what may have been denied by the insurance company and can be passed on to the patient (such as charges that have not reached the patient's deductible) are included in the patient's bill and collection efforts.

Customer Service

The final step in the revenue cycle is the customer service efforts of an organization. The key point here is that this function serves to resolve any errors or issues that may have happened in the previous steps. If, for example, a patient does not understand his or her bill, a good customer service system can help to reduce the delay in collection that this confusion can cause. Taking a day or two to return a patient's phone call may result in a significant delay in the collection process.

SHORT-TERM OBLIGATIONS

To this point, this chapter has focused on short-term resources. We now turn our attention to management of short-term obligations, or current liabilities. Careful management of such obligations can save a substantial amount of money. Some short-term obligations that need management attention are *accounts payable, payroll payable, notes payable,* and *taxes payable.*

Accounts payable represents amounts that the organization owes to its suppliers. *Payroll payable* is an amount owed to employees. *Notes payable* represents an obligation to repay money that has been borrowed. *Taxes payable* includes income, sales, real estate, payroll, and other taxes.

As a general rule, managers should try to delay payment of short-term obligations to keep resources in the organization available to earn interest, or to avoid unnecessary short-term borrowing and related interest expenses. However, this must be balanced

against any negative consequences related to delayed payments.

Accounts Payable

Accounts payable is often called *trade credit.* In most cases, there is no interest charge for trade credit, assuming that payment is made when due. For example, Keepuwell might order and receive a shipment of syringes. Shortly afterward, it receives an invoice from the supplier. The invoice generally has a due date.

Some suppliers charge interest for payments received after the due date. Others do not. A common practice in many industries is to offer a discount for prompt payment. On an invoice, under a heading called *terms,* there may be an indication such as: 2/10 N/30. This would be read as "two ten, net thirty." A discount of 2/10 N/30 means that if payment is received within 10 days of the invoice date, the payer can take a 2% discount off the total. If payment is not made within 10 days, then the full amount of the bill is due 30 days from the invoice date. Some companies state their terms in relation to the end of the month. Terms of 2/10 EOM (two ten, end of month) mean that the buyer can take a 2% discount for payments received by the company no later than 10 days after the end of the month in which the invoice is issued.

One confusing element is that if you don't take the early payment discount, you pay the "net" amount, which is the full amount on the invoice. Usually, *net* refers to a number after a subtraction has been made. The reason for this strange terminology is that many times organizations negotiate a discount from the full price at the time an order is placed. For example, suppose that the regular wholesale price for tongue depressors is $24.00 per box. However, Keepuwell successfully negotiated a 20% discount off the official or "list" price. Perhaps this is a volume discount. Alternatively, it may be a discount that the manufacturer offers to meet a competitor's price. From the seller's viewpoint, $24.00 is the list or *gross price*, $20.00 is the invoice or *net price*, and $19.60 is the net price less a discount for prompt payment (the $20.00 negotiated price less the 2% discount = $19.60).

Does it make sense to take advantage of discounts for prompt payment? A formula can be used to determine the annual interest rate implicit in trade credit discounts:

$$\text{Implicit Interest Rate} = \frac{\text{Discount}}{\text{Discounted Price}} \times \frac{\text{365 Days}}{\text{Days Sooner}} \times 100\%$$

For example, suppose that Keepuwell purchased $10,000 of pharmaceutical supplies with payment terms of 2/10 N/30. A 2% discount on a $10,000 purchase is $200. This means that if the discount is taken, only $9,800 has to be paid. By taking the discount, Keepuwell must make payment by the 10th day rather than the 30th day. This means that payment is made 20 days sooner than would otherwise be the case.

$$\text{Implicit Interest Rate} = \frac{\$200}{\$9,800} \times \frac{\text{365 Days}}{\text{20 Days}} \times 100\% = 37.2\%$$

Although the stated discount rate of 2% seems to be rather small, it is actually quite large on an annualized basis. Gaining a 2% discount in exchange for paying just twenty days sooner represents a high annual rate of return. Suppose that the organization had $9,800 of cash available to pay the bill promptly and take the discount. In order for it to make sense not to pay the bill promptly and take the discount, it would have to invest the money for the next 20 days in an invest-

ment that would earn at least $200 over that period. Any investment that could give us that return would be earning profits at a rate of at least 37.2% per year. Because most organizations do not have access to short-term investments that are assured of earning such a high rate, it pays to take the discount and pay promptly. Even if you have to borrow money to take the discount you should, as long as you can borrow at an interest rate of less than 37.2% per year.

This assumes, of course, that the invoice will be paid on time if the discount is not taken. Suppose, however, that Keepuwell often pays its bills late. Sometimes, it pays after 3 months. Would it make sense to take the discount and pay in 10 days, or to wait and pay the bill after 90 days? Paying after 10 days is 80 days earlier than if we normally wait for 90 days before making our payment.

$$\text{Implicit Interest Rate} = \frac{\text{Discount}}{\text{Discounted Price}} \times \frac{\text{365 Days}}{\text{Days Sooner}} \times 100\%$$

$$\text{Implicit Interest Rate} = \frac{\$200}{\$9,800} \times \frac{\text{365 Days}}{\text{80 Days}} \times 100\% = 9.3\%$$

If Keepuwell can earn more than 9.3% on its investments, or if Keepuwell does not have enough money to pay the bill and a bank would charge more than 9.3% to lend the money, then Keepuwell is better off waiting. However, that assumes its suppliers are willing to wait and will not charge interest for late payments. Otherwise, Keepuwell should pay promptly and take the discount.

Excel Template

Use Template 19 to calculate the implicit interest rate for any discount for prompt payment. The template is on the Web at www.jbpub.com.

Payroll Payable

Each organization must decide upon a number of general policies, such as how many holidays, vacation days, and sick days employees get. Most new organizations are well advised to be fairly conservative to start. It is much easier to later decide that you can afford to give employees more vacation than it is to reduce the vacation allowance. The benefits of employee morale from a more liberal policy must be weighed against the cost of paying for days not worked.

Another policy decision relates to whether employees will receive pay for sick days in cash if they do not use them. If employees are allowed to accumulate sick days and know they will get paid eventually whether they take them or not, then they are more likely to accumulate a substantial bank of sick leave for a serious illness. When sick leave is lost each year if it is not used, employees are more likely to take sick days when they are not sick. This encourages a culture whereby employees lie to the organization.

Although it is costly to pay employees for accumulated sick leave, it is important to bear in mind that for many employees it will be years or decades before that payment is made. In the intervening time, the employer has had the benefit of earning interest on the money. If sick leave can't be accumulated, most of it will be used and paid for currently. So it may actually turn out to be less costly to allow accumulation than to enforce a "use it or lose it" policy.

Each organization must also decide on the length of the payroll period, and how soon payment is made to employees once the payroll period ends. Employees could be paid daily, weekly, biweekly, or monthly. They could be paid on the last day of the payroll period, or a few days or a week later. The less frequently you pay, the fewer checks that must be written, reducing bookkeeping costs. Further, paying less frequently and later means that the employer holds onto the cash for a longer period, earning more interest. On the other hand, employees obviously prefer to be paid more often and sooner. Poor morale can turn out to be more costly than the benefits that the organization may have accrued in the form of extra interest.

Payroll policy must also focus on other *fringe benefits.* The organization must decide what benefits to offer, and how much will be paid by the employer versus the portion paid by the employee. Other fringes (in addition to vacation, holidays, and sick leave) include items such as health and dental insurance, life insurance, child care, car allowances, parking, and pensions.

Accounting and Compliance Issues

Payroll accounting is complicated by the various deductions that must be made from wages. The most prominent reason for payroll deductions relates to tax compliance issues. It is necessary to withhold income taxes, Social Security (FICA) taxes, unemployment insurance, and disability insurance. Most states also have state income taxes that must be withheld, and some localities have payroll or income taxes.

Calculating taxes can be complicated. At times the government changes the tax rates or the amount of income subject to tax. It is also critical to submit payments to the various governments on a timely basis. We don't want to pay early, because we are better off holding the money in our interest-bearing account for as long as possible. On the other hand, there are costly penalties for late payment that should be avoided.

In addition to taxes and other government-required deductions, there are a number of other types of deductions from payroll. These include amounts for health and dental insurance, pensions, life insurance, and other similar items. Often the employer pays for part or most of these benefits, and the employee makes a lesser contribution. Payroll can be further complicated if your organization pays bonuses, overtime, or piecework pay.

It is probably inadvisable for nonfinancial managers to attempt to take on too much of the payroll process themselves. Either the organization needs to have a payroll department that can specialize in this process, or an outside payroll vendor should be used. Each organization must determine whether it is best to prepare the payroll in house or to use a service. At least part of this analysis must rest on:

- the relative cost of preparing the payroll internally versus using a service;
- a determination of whether the company has the expertise to be able to prepare payroll internally; and
- whether the organization's employees have the time to prepare the payroll internally.

Suppose that you decide to use an outside service. That doesn't mean that your company will have nothing left to do. First, all payroll changes, such as newly hired employees or raises, must be carefully recorded. Second, employees need to be clearly classified between professional staff, hourly employees, commission-based, and piecework employees. Finally, your company must accurately record hours worked, sales, or other key information needed to calculate wages earned.

Notes Payable

Notes payable are short-term loans evidenced by a written document signed by all parties that specifies the amount borrowed, the interest rate, and the due date for repayment. Often such notes are *demand notes*. This means that the lender has the right to call for immediate payment of the full amount borrowed, plus accrued interest, at any time.

The interest on a note or loan is equal to the amount of the loan, multiplied by the annual interest rate, multiplied by the fraction of the year that the loan is outstanding:

$$\text{Interest} = \text{Loan Amount} \times \text{Interest Rate per Year} \times \text{Fraction of Year}$$

For example, the interest on a 6%, 6-month note for $25,000 is:

$$\text{Interest} = \$25,000 \times 6\% \times \tfrac{1}{2} = \$750$$

Typically, organizations obtain short-term debt by borrowing money from banks using *unsecured* notes. An unsecured note has no specific asset that will be delivered to the lender if the borrower fails to make required payments (*collateral*). A secured note is one that has collateral. If the borrower fails to repay an unsecured loan, the lender joins with all other creditors in making a general claim on the resources of the organization. This is riskier than having collateral; unsecured loans, therefore, often have higher interest rates to offset the lender's higher risk.

For organizations that have limited financial resources, another approach for obtaining short-term financing is to borrow money from an organization that specializes in financing and factoring receivables. A *factoring* arrangement is one in which we sell our receivables. The buyer is called a *factor*. The right to collect those receivables then belongs to the factor. In most cases, if receivables are factored, the organization receives less than it would have received, but gets the cash sooner. Alternatively, a financing arrangement is one whereby money is borrowed with the receivables being used as collateral in case we cannot repay the loan.

Taxes Payable

Taxes payable represents a short-term obligation. As with other short-term obligations, these should not be paid before they are due. However, because there are often penalties in addition to interest for the late payment, managers must have a system in place to ensure that taxes are paid on time.

BANKING RELATIONSHIPS

Working capital management often requires a good working relationship with one or more banks. A system of checking and savings accounts is required by most organizations. Many short-term investments are made with one of the organization's banks. And, of course, money is often borrowed from banks.

Many people think of banks as a place to go when you need a loan. However, you are much more likely to get a loan if you establish a long-term relationship with a bank. Let the bank get to know your organization. Use the bank for some of your investment needs. Teach the bank about the cyclical patterns in your organization that are likely to generate cash surpluses at some times of the year and cash deficits at other times.

It is important to be able to show banks that your organization has thought through its working capital situation. How much money do you expect to borrow over the next year? When? What for? How long will you need the money? Banks are more likely to lend to organizations that can anticipate temporary cash needs long before the cash is needed, especially if you can show when you expect to be able to repay the loan.

Some organizations borrow specific amounts on short-term *commercial* loans. Such loans, often called *commercial paper,* were discussed in the short-term investment section of this chapter. If your needs are intermediate-term, then a *term* loan, typically from 1 to 5 years, can be arranged. Such commercial loans and term loans can be arranged at the time the money is needed. However, many organizations arrange for a line of bank credit at a time when they currently have more than adequate cash.

For example, Keepuwell Clinic might arrange for a $1 million line of credit at the bank where it handles most of its routine financial transactions. The arrangement typically includes repayment terms and interest rates tied to some benchmark rate that may vary over time. The *prime rate* is the interest rate banks charge their most creditworthy clients. Keepuwell Clinic might negotiate for a loan at 2% over prime (referred to as 2 *OP*) at a time when the prime rate is 6%. Suppose that Keepuwell doesn't need to borrow any of its $1 million credit line for 6 months. At the time the prime has fallen to 5.5%. The interest rate on money borrowed against the line of credit would be 7.5%, which is 2% over the then-current prime. If the prime rate changes again, the interest rate on the outstanding portion of the loan changes as well. A common alternative to the prime rate, especially for companies with international operations, is the London Interbank Offered Rate (LIBOR). The LIBOR rate represents the rate that banks charge each other in the London Eurocurrency market. Having a credit line allows the organization to hold lower cash reserves than it might otherwise need.

In exchange for credit arrangements, many times banks require an organization to keep *compensating balances* in the bank. That is, the organization must always keep a certain amount of money in the bank. Why agree to a compensating balance arrangement? Because the line of credit greatly exceeds the compensating balance and provides a level of cash safety that the organization might not otherwise have. Will the bank make a loan to your organization, or offer it a line of credit? The bank looks for things such as positive cash flow from your operations, a strong management team, and adequate collateral. The weaker your position in these areas, the higher the rate of interest charged. If you are too weak, the bank will not make the loan.

However, this is a two-way street. You don't want to borrow from just any bank. You need to pick the right bank for you. You need a big enough bank to meet all your needs, but not such a big bank that you are irrelevant to them. You need a bank that has experience serving health care organizations. Such a bank better understands your problems and needs. Does your organization have international operations? If so, you may want to chose a bank that has an international department. You need a bank with a range of services to meet your needs now and as your organization grows. Banks can be useful in many ways, sometimes offering advice on how to run your organization better, or even linking you with potential customers.

Concentration Banking

Although many organizations deal with more than one bank, they often maintain a significant presence at one or more banks, which are referred to as *concentration banks*. Arrangements can be made with the concentration bank to *sweep* or transfer money into and out of accounts automatically.

For example, suppose that a nationwide chain of drugstores has many individual locations around the country that collect cash from customers and deposit that cash in local banks. The company wants to have access to those deposits to make disbursements for various purposes. An arrangement may be made in which the concentration bank transfers balances from these other feeder accounts to a master account at the concentration bank. There could be daily, weekly, or monthly transfers, depending on the expected balances in the accounts.

The process can also be reversed with *zero-balance accounts*. An organization can write checks on an account that has a zero balance. When the checks are presented for payment, the bank keeps a tally of the total amount disbursed. That amount is then automatically transferred from one central account at the concentration bank into the zero-balance account.

This type of automatic transferring of funds back and forth allows the organization to have quicker access to its cash resources for payment needs. It also allows it to maintain less cash in total than it would if it had cash balances in many different accounts. The excess cash can be invested and may enable the organization to earn a higher yield on investments by purchasing securities in larger denominations.

KEY CONCEPTS

Working capital management—Management of short-term resources and short-term obligations to maximize financial results.

Short-term resource management:

Cash is kept for transactions, safety, and investment opportunities.

Short-term investments—Bank deposits, CDs, money market funds, T-bills, unsecured notes, commercial paper, repurchase agreements (repos), and similar securities.

Accounts receivable aging schedule—Management report that shows how long receivables have been outstanding.

Inventory management—Inventory levels should be kept as low as possible, while allowing for adequate inventory for current use and as a safety measure.

a. *Economic order quantity* (EOQ)— Technique used to calculate the optimal amount of inventory to purchase at one time.

b. *Just-in-time* (JIT)—Inventory management approach that calls for the arrival of inventory just as it is needed, resulting in zero inventory levels.

Revenue Cycle Management—Management of the all processes associated with generating revenue and converting to cash. Begins with data gathering at time of scheduling and runs through customer care services and problem resolution.

Short-term obligation management:

Trade credit and terms—Payables to suppliers. Terms represent the payment agreement, sometimes including a discount for prompt payment.

Payroll payable—Amount owed to employees. Payroll policy must consider payroll benefits as well as when and how often payroll is paid.

Notes payable—Short-term loans that may be unsecured or secured by collateral.

Banking relationships—Needed for transactions (e.g., checking), short-term investments, and borrowing.

Concentration bank—Bank where an organization keeps a significant presence.

Short-term loans—Commercial loans, term loans, and lines of credit. The interest rate may be a specific set rate, or may vary with a benchmark such as the prime rate.

Compensating balances—Balances that must be maintained on deposit at all times in exchange for a line of credit (prearranged loan to be made when and if needed in an amount up to an agreed upon limit).

TEST YOUR KNOWLEDGE

See www.jbpub.com/catalog/0763726753/supplements.htm.

CHAPTER 15

Investment Analysis: What Should We Do Next?

Analysis of investments in long-term projects is referred to as *capital budgeting*. Long-term projects are worthy of special attention because they frequently require large initial investments and because the cash outlay to start projects often precedes the receipt of cash inflows by a significant period of time. In such cases, we are interested in being able to predict the profitability of the project. We want to be sure that the profits from the project are greater than what we could have received from alternative investments or uses of our money.

This chapter focuses on how managers can evaluate long-term projects and determine whether the expected return from the projects is great enough to justify taking the risks that are inherent in long-term investments. Several different approaches to capital budgeting are discussed: the payback method, the net present value method, and the internal rate of return method. The latter two of these methods require us to acknowledge the implication of the "time value of money."

The *time value of money* refers to the fact that money received at different points in time is not equally valuable. To give a rather elementary example, suppose that you are in pharmaceutical sales and someone offered to buy your product for $250, and they

are willing to pay you either today or 1 year from today. You will certainly prefer to receive the $250 today. At the very least, you could put the $250 in a bank and earn interest in the intervening year.

Suppose, however, that the buyer offered you $250 today or $330 in 22 months. Now your decision is much more difficult. How sure are you that the individual will pay you 22 months from now? Perhaps he or she will be bankrupt by then. What could we do with the money if we received it today? Would we put the $250 in some investment that would yield us more than $330 22 months from today? These are questions that we have to be able to answer to evaluate long-term investment opportunities. But first let's discuss some basic issues of investment analysis.

INVESTMENT OPPORTUNITIES

The first step that must be taken in investment analysis is to identify the investment opportunity. Such opportunities fall into two major classes: new project investments and replacement or reinvestment in existing projects. New project ideas can come from a variety of sources. They may be the result of research and development activity or exploration. Some health care organizations, like pharmaceutical companies, have departments solely devoted to new product development. Ideas may come from outside of the organization. Reinvestment is often the result of managers pointing out that certain equipment needs to be replaced. Such replacement should not be automatic. If a substantial outlay is required, it may be an appropriate time to reevaluate the product or project to determine if the profits being generated and services being provided are adequate to justify continued additional investment.

DATA GENERATION

The data needed to evaluate an investment opportunity are the expected cash flows related to the investment. Many projects have a large initial cash outflow as we acquire plant and equipment and incur start-up costs prior to actual production and sale of our new product or delivery of our new service. In the years that follow, there will be receipt of cash from the sale of our product (or service) and there will be cash expenditures related to the expenses of production. The difference between the cash inflows and cash outflows each year represent the net cash flows for the year.

You're probably wondering why we have started this discussion with cash flow instead of net income for each year. There are several important reasons. First, net income or the increase in net assets, even if it were a perfect measure of profitability, doesn't consider the time value of money. For instance, suppose that we have two alternative projects. The first project requires that we purchase a machine for $20,000 in cash. The machine has a 10-year useful life. Depreciation expense is $2,000 per year.

A totally different project requires that we lease a machine for $2,000 a year for 10 years, with lease payments at the start of each

year. Are the two alternative projects equal? No, they aren't. Even though they both have an expense of $2,000 per year for 10 years, one project requires us to spend $20,000 at the beginning. The other project requires an outlay of only $2,000 in the first year. In this second project, we could hold on to $18,000 that had been spent right away in the first project. That $18,000 can be invested and can earn additional profits for the firm before the next lease payment is due.

The data needed for investment or project analysis includes cash flow information for each of the years of the investment's life. Naturally, we cannot be 100% certain about how much the project will cost and how much we will eventually receive. There is no perfect solution for the fact that we have to make estimates. However, we must be aware at all times that, because our estimates may not be fully correct, there is an element of risk. Project analysis must be able to assess whether the expected return can compensate for the risks we are taking. It should also include consideration of any taxes that will have to be paid.

THE PAYBACK METHOD

The payback method of analysis evaluates projects based on how long it takes to recover the amount of money put into the project. The shorter the payback period, the better. Certainly there is some intuitive appeal to this method. The sooner we get our money out of the project, the lower the risk. If we have to wait a number of years for a project to "pay off," all kinds of things can go wrong. Furthermore, given high interest rates, the longer we have our initial investment tied up, the more costly it is for us.

Table 15-1 presents an example of the payback method: four alternative projects are compared. In each project, the initial outlay is $8,000. By the end of 2009, projects one and two have recovered the initial $8,000 investment. Therefore they have a payback period of 3 years. Projects three and four do not recover the initial investment until the end of 2010. Their payback period is 4 years, and they are therefore considered to be inferior to the other two projects.

It is not difficult at this point to see one of the principal weaknesses of the payback method. It ignores what happens after the payback period. The total cash flow for project four is much greater than the cash received from any of the other projects. In a situation in which cash flows extend for 20 or 30 years, this problem might not be as obvious, but it could cause us to choose incorrectly.

Is that the only problem with this method? No. Another obvious problem stems from the fact that according to this method, projects one and two are equally attractive because they both have a 3-year payback period. Although their total cash flows are the same, the timing is different. Project one provides $1 in 2008, and then $7,999 in 2009. Project two generates $7,999 in 2008 and only $1 in 2009. Are these two projects equally as good because their total cash flows are the same? *No.* The extra $7,998 received in 2008 from project two is available for investment in other profitable opportunities for 1 extra year as compared to project one. Therefore, project two is clearly superior to project one. The problem is that the payback method doesn't formally take into account the time value of money.

This deficiency is obvious when looking at project three as well. Project three appears to be less valuable than projects one or two on two counts. First, its payback is 4 years rather than 3, and second, its total cash flow is less than either project one or two. But if we consider the time value of money, then project three is better than either project one or two. With project three, we get the $7,999 right away. The earnings on that $7,999 during 2008 and 2009 will more than offset the shorter payback and larger cash flow of projects one and two.

Although payback is commonly used for a quick and dirty project evaluation, problems associated with the payback method are quite serious. There are several methods, commonly referred to as *discounted cash flow models*, that overcome these problems. Elsewhere in this chapter, we discuss the more commonly used of these methods, namely, *net present value* and *internal rate of return.* However, before we discuss them, we need to specifically

Table 15-1   Payback Method—Alternative Projects

| | Project Cash Flows | | | |
	One	Two	Three	Four
January 2007	$ (8,000)	$ (8,000)	$ (8,000)	$ (8,000)
January 1, 2007–December 31, 2007	0	0	7,999	7,000
January 1, 2008–December 31, 2008	1	7,999	0	999
January 1, 2009–December 31, 2009	7,999	1	0	0
January 1, 2010–December 31, 2010	10,000	10,000	10,000	100,000
Total	$10,000	$10,000	$ 9,999	$ 99,999
Payback Period	3 Years	3 Years	4 Years	4 Years

consider the issues and mechanics surrounding time value of money calculations.

TIME VALUE OF MONEY

It is very easy to think of projects in terms of total dollars of cash received. Unfortunately, this tends to be misleading. Consider a project in which we invest $8,000 and in return we receive $10,400 after 3 years. We have made a cash profit of $2,400. Because the profit was earned over a 3-year period, it is a profit of $800 per year. Because $800 is 10% of the initial $8,000 investment, we have apparently earned a 10% return on our money. Although this is true, that 10% is calculated based on simple interest.

Consider putting money into a bank that pays a 10% return "compounded annually." *Compounded annually* means that the bank calculates interest at the end of each year and adds the interest to the entire amount on deposit. In future years, interest is earned not only on the initial deposit, but also on interest earned in prior years.

If we put $8,000 in the bank at 10% compounded annually we would earn $800 of interest in the first year. At the beginning of the second year our principal plus interest is $8,800. For the second year, the interest on the $8,800 is $880. At the beginning of the third year, we have $9,680 (the $8,000 initial deposit plus the $800 interest from the first year, plus the $880 interest from the second year). The interest for the third year is $968. We, therefore, have a total of $10,648 at the end of the 3 years.

Table 15-2 lays out the interest earnings from our hypothetical investment using both the simple interest calculations and the compound interest calculations. The 10% interest compounded annually gives a different result from the 10% simple interest. We have $10,648 instead of $10,400 from the project. The reason for this difference is the fact that with compound interest we earn interest on our interest.

In our example above, we have not felt the full power of compound interest. Take a slightly different example: In 1624 the Dutch purchased New York from the Native Americans who inhabited Manhattan Island for $24 in gold medallions. If the Native Americans had invested the $24 worth of gold in a venture that earned 10% simple interest for the last 383 years (from 1624 to 2007) they would now have an investment worth $943.20 ($24 plus $2.40 of interest per year for 383 years). On the other hand, if they had invested the $24 in a venture that earned 10% compounded annually, they would now have an investment worth

Table 15-2   Comparison of Simple Interest and Compound Interest

	Simple Interest			Compound Interest		
	Principal Balance	Interest Earned	Cumulative Balance	Principal Balance	Interest Earned	Cumulative Balance
Year 1	$ 8,000	$ 800	$ 8,800	$ 8,000	$ 800	$ 8,800
Year 2	8,000	800	9,600	8,800	880	9,680
Year 3	8,000	800	10,400	9,680	968	10,648
TOTAL		$ 2,400			$ 2,648	

$171,241,749,947,654,000! That is an amount well in excess of the annual United States' Gross Domestic Product. And the result is substantially greater if earnings are compounded quarterly or monthly! Obviously, this example is a bit extreme, but the point is that compounding and the time value of money is an extremely important aspect of the analysis of long-term projects, particularly if they have monthly compounding, which is often the case.

There are some standard terms and approaches to calculating compound interest. Consider a cash amount of $100 today. We refer to it as a *present value* (PV or P). How much could this cash amount accumulate to if we invested it at an interest rate (i) or rate of return (r) of 10% for a period of time (N) of 2 years? Assuming that we compound annually, the $100 earns $10 in the first year (10% of $100). This $10 is added to the $100. In the second year our $110 earns $11 (that is, 10% of $110). The future value (FV or F) is $121. That is, 2 years into the future we have $121.

Mechanically this is a simple process—multiply the interest rate times the initial investment to find the interest for the first period. Add the interest to the initial investment. Then multiply the interest rate times the initial investment. Then multiply the interest rate times the initial investment plus all interest already accumulated to find the interest for the second year.

Although this is not complicated, it can be rather tedious. To simplify this process, mathematical formulas have been developed to solve a variety of "time value of money" problems. The most basic of these formulas states that:

$$FV = PV(1 + i)^N$$

This formula and the others that follow have been built into both business calculators and computer spreadsheet programs. If we supply the appropriate raw data, the calculator or spreadsheet software performs all of the necessary interest computations.

For instance, if we wanted to know what $100 would grow to in 2 years at 10%, we would simply tell our calculator that the present value, P or PV (depending on the brand of calculator you use), equals $100; the interest rate, %i or r, equals 10%; and the number of periods, N, equals 2. Then we would ask the calculator to compute F or FV, the future value.

Can we use this method if compounding occurs more frequently than once a year? Bonds often pay interest twice a year. Banks often compound monthly to calculate mortgage payments. Using our example of $100 invested for 2 years at 10%, we could easily adjust the calculation for semiannual, quarterly, or monthly compounding. For example, for semiannual compounding, N becomes 4 because there are two semiannual periods per year for 2 years. The rate of return, or interest rate, becomes 5%. If the rate earned is 10% for a full year, then it is half of that, or 5%, for each half year.

For quarterly compounding, N equals 8 (four quarters per year for 2 years) and i equals 2.5% (10% per year divided by four quarters per year). For monthly compounding, N equals 24 and i equals 10%/12. Thus, for monthly compounding, we tell the calculator that $PV = 100, $i = 10\%/12$, and $N = 24$. Then we tell the calculator to compute FV. We need a calculator designed to perform present value functions to do this.

If we expect to receive $121 in 2 years, can we calculate how much that is worth today? This question calls for a reversal of the compounding process. Suppose we expect to earn a return on our money of 10%. What we are really asking here is, "How much would we have to invest today at 10% to get

$121 in 2 years?" The answer requires unraveling compound interest. If we calculate how much of the $121 to be received in 2 years is interest earned on our original investment, then we know the present value of that $121. This process of removing or unraveling the interest is called *discounting*. The 10% rate is referred to as a *discount rate*. Using the calculator, this is a simple process. We again supply the *i* and the *N*, but instead of telling the calculator the *PV* and asking for the *FV*, we tell it the *FV* and ask it to calculate the *PV*.

We posited a problem of whether to accept $250 today or $330 in 22 months. Assume that we can invest money in a project with a 10% return and monthly compounding. Which choice is better? We can tell our calculator (by the way, if you have access to a business-oriented calculator, you can work out these calculations as we go) that *FV* = $330, *N* = 22, and *i* = 10%/12. If we then ask it to compute *PV*, we find that the present value is $275. This means that if we invest $275 today at 10% compounded monthly for 22 months, it accumulates to $330. That is, receiving $330 in 22 months is equivalent to having $275 today. Because this amount is greater than $250, our preference is to wait for the money, assuming there is no risk of default. Looking at this problem another way, how much would our $250 grow to if we invested it for 22 months at 10%? Here we have *PV* = $250, *N* = 22, and *i* = 10%/12. Our calculation indicates that the *FV* = $300. If we wait, we have $330 22 months from now. If we take $250 today and invest it at 10%, we only have $300 22 months from now. We find that we are better off waiting for the $330, assuming we are sure that we will receive it.

Are we limited to solving for only the present or future value? No, this methodology is quite flexible. Assume, for example, that we wish to put $100,000 aside today to pay off a $1,000,000 loan in 15 years. What rate of return must be earned, compounded annually, for our $100,000 to grow to $1,000,000? Here we have the present value, or $100,000; the number of periods, 15 years; and the future value, or $1,000,000. It is a simple process to determine the required rate of return. If we simply supply our calculator with the *PV*, *FV*, and *N*, the calculator readily supplies the *i*, which is 16.6% in this case.

Or, for that matter, if we had $100,000 today and knew that we could earn a 13% return, we could calculate how long it would take to accumulate $1,000,000. Here we know *PV*, *FV*, and *i*, and we wish to find *N*. In this case, *N* = 18.8 years. Given any three of our four basic components, *PV*, *FV*, *N*, and *i*, we can solve for the fourth. This is because the calculator is simply using our basic formula stated earlier and solving for the missing variable.

So, far, however, we have considered only a single payment. Suppose that we don't have $100,000 today, but we are willing to put $10,000 aside every year for 15 years. If we earn 12%, will we have enough to repay $1,000,000 at the end of the 15 years? There are two ways to solve this problem. We can determine the future value, 15 years from now, of each of the individual payments. We would have to do 15 separate calculations because each succeeding payment earns interest for 1 year less. We then have to sum the future value of each of the payments. This is rather tedious. A second way to solve this problem is by using a formula that accumulates the payments for us. The formula is:

$$FV = PMT \left[\frac{(1+i)^N - 1}{i} \right]$$

In this formula, *PMT* represents the payment made each period, or annuity payment. Although you may think of annuities as payments made once a year, an annuity simply means payments that are exactly the same in amount, and are made at equally spaced intervals of time, such as monthly, quarterly, or annually. For example, mortgage payments of $321.48 per month represent an annuity.

To solve problems with a series of identical payments, we have five variables instead of four. We now have *FV, PV, N, i,* and *PMT.* However, *PV* doesn't appear in our formula. There is a separate formula that relates present value to a series of payments. This formula is:

$$FV = PMT \left[\frac{1 - \frac{1}{(1 + i)^N}}{i} \right]$$

Annuity formulas are built into business calculators and computer spreadsheet programs such as Excel or Lotus 123. With the spreadsheet program or calculator, you can easily solve for *PV, i, N,* or *PMT,* if you have the other three variables. Similarly, you can solve for *FV, i, N,* or *PMT* given the other three. For instance, how much would we pay monthly on a 20-year mortgage at 12% if we borrowed $50,000? The *PV* is $50,000, the interest rate (%*i*) is 1% per month, and the number of months (*N*) is 240. Given these three factors, we can solve for the annuity payment (*PMT*). It is $551 per month.

Annuity formulas provide you with a basic framework for solving many problems concerning receipt or payment of cash in different time periods. Keep in mind that the annuity method can be used only if the amount of the payment is the same each period. If that isn't the case, each payment must be evaluated separately.

Using Microsoft Excel

Most computer spreadsheet programs have the capability to do time value of money calculations built right into the program. To make use of these features, the user only needs to understand the basics of time value of money and to know how to access the built-in functions of the spreadsheet. Microsoft Excel has become the most widely used computer spreadsheet program, so we demonstrate some standard time value of money calculations using Microsoft Excel as an example. Other spreadsheet applications may differ slightly, but should function in much the same way as Excel.

Step 1: Identify the Components of the Calculation

Like any time value of money problem, the first step to finding the solution is to clearly identify what you are solving for and all the information, such as interest rate and number of periods, that you already know. Take our example from earlier in the chapter. We have $100 today (the *PV*) and we want to know how much it will accumulate to (*FV*) over 2 years (the number of periods or *N* or *nper*) at 10% (the interest rate, or *i* or *rate*). As you may recall, the accumulation, or future value, when we did this example earlier came out to be $121. In this example we have identified what we are solving for—the *FV*. We have also identified all the other information we already know: *PV* = $100, *N* = 2, and *i* = 10%.

Step 2: Use the Appropriate Excel Function to Solve

The next step in using Excel to solve this problem is to "call" the appropriate function and insert the information we gathered in step 1. Calling the appropriate function is a simple matter of clicking on the Function Wizard button "*fx*" located on the tool bar. Figure 15-1 shows the location of the function wizard.

Our example is a future value problem. After clicking on the Function Wizard *fx*, an "Insert Function" window opens. We now

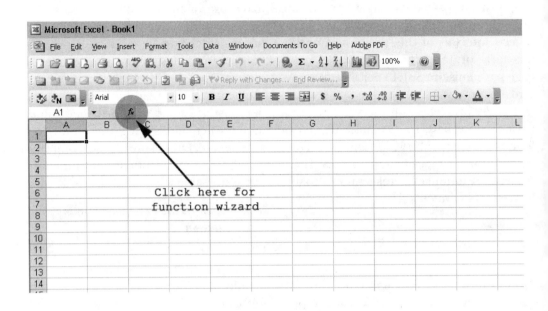

Figure 15-1 Location of the Function Wizard

need to specify that we are interested in the *FV* function. The time value of money functions are categorized as "financial" functions. Selecting the financial functions "category" opens a list of functions that includes *FV* as one of the choices. Figure 15-2 shows the open function wizard and the selection of the financial category and FV function.

After clicking "OK" at the bottom of the Insert Function window, the future value "Function Arguments" window opens. The information gathered as step one can now be entered directly into each of the appropriate cells. Figure 15-3 shows the future value function window, which has been completed with the information from our example. You should note that the "Pmt" cell has a 0. This cell is the amount of annuity payments made in each of the periods. In our example we do not have any payments in the two periods, but rather have an upfront payment of $100 (the *PV*). It should also be noted that payments, or cash

outflows, are listed as negative numbers. Also, it is essential that the interest rate be shown either as .10 or as 10%. If you simply use 10 for the rate, you get an incorrect result. Finally, the window displays the result of the calculation near the bottom of the function window.

In our example, we entered the data for the calculation directly into the function wizard. The data can also be entered into the wizard by linking to data already in the spreadsheet. Figure 15-4 shows the same problem using data in the spreadsheet to populate the function wizard.

The use of Excel is not limited to future value calculations. Figure 15-5 shows the present value function for another problem presented earlier in the chapter. In this example, the future value is $330, the number of periods is 22 months, and the interest rate is 10% per month (.10/12). The solution of $275 is the present value of $330 22 months from now.

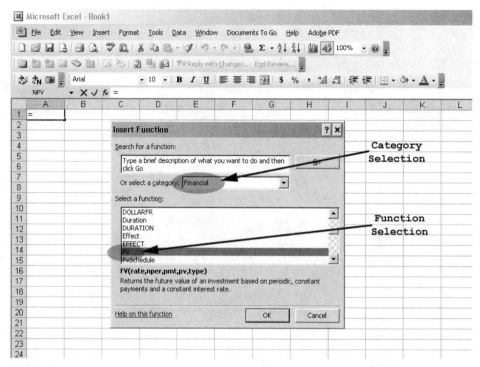

Figure 15-2 Category and Function Selection

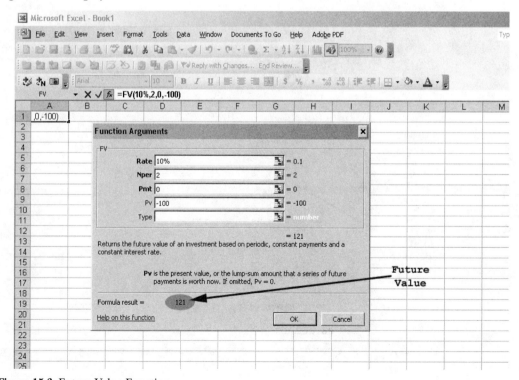

Figure 15-3 Future Value Function

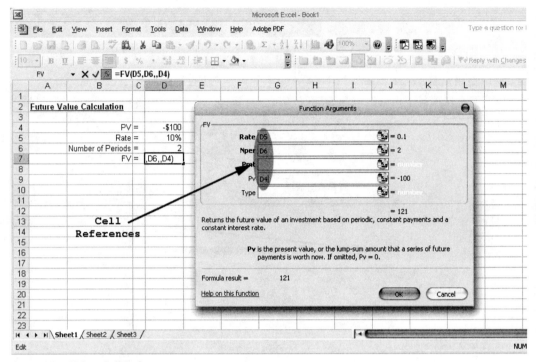

Figure 15-4 Using Cell References

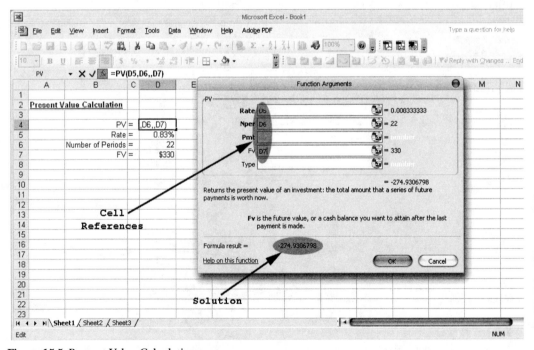

Figure 15-5 Present Value Calculation

With a solid understanding of how to calculate the changing value of money over time, we can now turn our attention to the different analytic methods used for evaluating long-term projects. Taken together, these approaches are called *discounted cash flow* methods. They are all premised on the fact that the time value of money has a significant impact on the evaluation of different project cash flows.

THE NET PRESENT VALUE METHOD

The net present value (NPV) method of analysis determines whether a project earns more or less than a stated desired rate of return. The starting point of the analysis is determination of this rate.

The Hurdle Rate

The rate of return required for a project to be acceptable is called the *required rate of return* or the *hurdle rate*. An acceptable project should be able to hurdle over—that is, be higher than—this rate.

The rate must take into account two key factors. First, we require a base profit to compensate for investing money in the project. We have a variety of opportunities for which we could use our money. We need to be paid a profit for foregoing the use of our money in some alternative venture. The second element concerns risk. Any time we enter a new investment, there is an element of risk. Perhaps the project won't work out exactly as expected. The project may turn out to be a failure. We have to be paid for being willing to undertake these risks. The two elements taken together determine our hurdle rate.

Although it is true that not-for-profit health care organizations often focus on the provision of service rather than profits, it is still critical that new ventures and new projects generate profits/surpluses. As discussed, profits generate the resources needed for replacement and reinvestment. In addition, when taking on a new venture or project, we do not want this activity to be a drain on the existing services of the organization. Therefore, we still need new projects to generate a certain level of profit so as not to harm the financial health of the organization. At a minimum, if a project is going to lose money, we must know that explicitly. Then we can make a choice: If we feel the services from the project are so important that we should do the project even if it loses money, then we must determine where the money will come from to subsidize the project.

There is no unique, standard required rate of return that is used by all health care organizations. Different sectors of the health care industry tend to have different base rates of return. For-profit pharmaceutical companies have very different required rates of return than community clinics. Further, within the various sectors of the health care system, one organization may have some advantage over other organizations (e.g., economies of scale) that allow it to have a higher base return. On top of that, different organizations, and even different projects within the same organization, have different types and degrees of risk. For example, for most hospitals, replacing old hospital beds with new updated models involves much less risk than opening a new outpatient surgery center.

One of the most prevalent risks that organizations take is the loss of purchasing power. That is, price-level inflation makes our money less valuable over time. Suppose we could buy a TV for $100, but instead we invest that money in a new product or service. If the new product or service generates a surplus of $4 in a year when the inflation rate is 5%, we actually lost purchasing power during the year. It now costs us $105 to buy a new TV. In for-profit organizations, after-tax profits must be compared to the inflation rate. The $4 noted would actually be even less after taxes, resulting in additional loss of purchasing power. This means that in deciding if a project is worthwhile, we have to consider whether the rate of return is high enough to cover our after-tax loss of purchasing power due to inflation. In other words, if our $100 allows us to buy a TV set today, and we invest that money instead for 1 year at 4%, even though we may have $104 after 1 year, we have actually lost rather than made money if at that point in time we do not have enough to buy a TV set.

We must also consider a variety of risks associated with any new venture or project. What if the demand for outpatient surgery fails to materialize? What if those who come in for service are all low-income patients without health insurance? What if state or federal laws change regarding the specific reimbursements for our new service? In the case of pharmaceuticals or medical equipment manufacturers, what if no one buys our product? The specific types of risks faced by an organization depend on the sector of the health care system and the specific circumstance of the organization. If 1 out of every 10 projects is a complete failure, but the other 9 are successful, then the rate of return earned on the 9 successful products must be high enough to not only provide a return on their own investment, but also to allow us to recover the losses from the project that failed. The organization's past experience with projects like the one being evaluated should be a guide in determining the risk portion of the hurdle rate.

When we add the desired return to all of the risk factors, the total is the organization's hurdle rate. In most organizations, the top financial officers determine an appropriate hurdle rate or rates and inform nonfinancial managers that this hurdle rate must be anticipated for a project to receive approval. Therefore, you usually do not have to go through a calculation of the hurdle rate yourself.

NPV Calculations

Once we know our hurdle rate, we can use the NPV method to assess whether a project is acceptable. The NPV method compares the present value of a project's cash inflows to the present value of its cash outflows. If the present value of the inflows is greater than the outflows, then the project is profitable because it is earning a rate of return that is greater than the hurdle rate.

For example, suppose that a potential project for our organization requires an initial outlay of $100,000. We expect the project to produce a net cash flow (cash inflows less cash outflows) of $65,000 in each of the 2 years of the project's life. Suppose our hurdle rate is 18%. Is this project worthwhile?

The cash receipts total $130,000, which is a profit of $30,000 overall, or $15,000 per year on our $100,000 investment. Is that a compounded return of at least 18%? At first glance it would appear that the answer is "no" because $15,000 is only 15% of $100,000. However, we haven't left our full $100,000 invested for the full 2 years. Our positive cash flow at the end of the first year is $65,000. We are not only making $15,000 profit, but we are also getting back half ($50,000) of our original investment. During the second year, we earn $15,000 profit on a remaining investment of only $50,000. It is not simply how much money you get from the project, but when you get it that is important. In Table 15-3, the top half of the table lays out the cash flows associated with this project.

Table 15-3   Project Cash Flow and Net Present Value Calculation

	Initial Outlay	Year 1	Year 2	Total
Initial Outlay	$ (100,000)			$ (100,000)
Annual Net Cash Flow		$65,000	$65,000	130,000
Total Project Cash Flow	$ (100,000)	$65,000	$65,000	$ 30,000
Net Present Value Calculations	**$ (100,000)**			
	101,767	**Discounting**		
Net Present Value	**$ 1,767**			

The bottom half of Table 15-3 (the shaded portion) shows the calculation of the NPV. The present value of an annuity of $65,000 per year for 2 years at 18% is $101,767 ($PV$ = ?; PMT = $65,000; N = 2; i = 18%). The present value of the initial $100,000 outflow is simply $100,000 because it is paid at the start of the project. The NPV is the present value of the inflows, $101,767, less the present value of the outflows, $100,000, which is $1,767. This number is greater than zero, so the project does indeed yield a return greater than 18%, on an annually compounded basis.

It may not be intuitively clear why this method works, or indeed, that it works at all. However, consider making a deal with your friend who is a banker. You agree that you will put a sum of money into the bank. At the end of the first year, the banker adds 18% to your account and you then withdraw $65,000. At the end of year 2, the banker credits interest to the balance in your account at an 18% rate. You then withdraw $65,000, which is exactly the total in the account at that time. The account has a zero balance. You ask your friend how much you must deposit today to be able to make the two future withdrawals outlined above. He replies, "$101,767."

If we deposit $101,767, at an 18% rate, it earns $18,318 during the first year. This leaves a balance of $120,085 in the account. We then withdraw $65,000, leaving a balance of $55,085 for the start of the second year. During the second year, $55,085 earns interest of $9,915 at a rate of 18%. This means that the balance in the account is $65,000 at the end of the second year. We then withdraw that amount.

The point of this bank deposit example is that when we earlier solved for the present value of the two $65,000 inflows using a hurdle rate of 18%, we found PV to be $101,767. We were finding exactly the amount of money we would have to pay today to get two payments of $65,000 if we were to earn exactly 18%. If we can invest a smaller amount than $101,767, but still get $65,000 per year for each of the 2 years, we must be earning more than 18% because we are putting in less than would be needed to earn 18%, but are getting just as much out. Here, we invest $100,000, which is less than $101,767, so we are earning a rate of return greater than 18%.

Conversely, if the banker had told us to invest less than $100,000 (i.e., if the present value of the two payments of $65,000 each at 18% was less than $100,000), then it means that by paying $100,000 we were putting in more money than we would have to in order to earn 18%; therefore, we must be earning less than 18%.

The NPV method gets around the problems of the payback method. It considers the full project life and considers the time value of money. Clearly, however, you can see that it is more difficult than the payback method. Another problem with it is that you must determine the hurdle rate before you can do any project analysis. The next method we look at eliminates the need to have a hurdle rate before performing the analysis.

INTERNAL RATE OF RETURN METHOD

One of the objections to the NPV method is that it never indicates what rate of return a project is earning. We simply find out whether it is earning more or less than a specified hurdle rate. This creates problems when comparing projects, all of which have positive NPVs.

One conclusion that can be drawn from our NPV discussion is that when the NPV is greater than zero, we are earning more than our required rate of return. If the NPV is less than zero, then we are earning less than our required rate of return. If the NPV is zero, we must be earning exactly the hurdle rate. Therefore, if we want to determine the exact rate that a project earns, all we need to do is to set the NPV equal to zero. Because the NPV is the PV of the inflows less the PV of the outflows, or:

$$NPV = PV \text{ Inflows} - PV \text{ Outflows}$$

then when we set the NPV equal to zero,

$$0 = PV \text{ Inflows} - PV \text{ Outflows}$$

that is equivalent to:

$$PV \text{ Inflows} = PV \text{ Outflows.}$$

All we have to do to find the rate of return that the project actually earns, or the "internal rate of return" (IRR), is to find the interest rate at which this equation is true.

For example, consider our NPV project discussed earlier that requires a cash outlay of $100,000 and produces a net cash inflow of $65,000 per year for 2 years. The present value of the outflow is simply the $100,000 ($PV = \$100,000$) we pay today. The inflows represent a 2-year ($N = 2$) annuity of $65,000 ($PMT = \$65,000$) per year. By supplying our calculator with the PV, N, and PMT, we can simply find the i or r (IRR). In this case, we find that the IRR is 19.4%.

Variable Cash Flow

This calculation is simple for any business calculator that can handle time value of money, frequently called *discounted cash flow* (DCF) analysis. However, this problem is somewhat simplistic because it assumed that we would receive exactly the same cash inflow each year. In most capital budgeting problems, it is much more likely that the cash inflows from a project will change each year. Many business calculators are not sophisticated enough to determine the IRR if the cash flows are not the same each year. However, computer spreadsheet programs are able to do the calculation.

PROJECT RANKING

Often, we are faced with a situation in which there are more acceptable projects than the number that we can afford to finance. In this case, we wish to choose the best projects. A simple way to do this is to determine the IRR on each project and then to rank the projects from the project with the highest IRR to the one with the lowest. We then simply start by accepting projects with the highest IRR and go down the list until we either run out of money or reach our minimum acceptable rate of return.

In general, this approach allows an organization to optimize its overall rate of return. However, it is possible for this approach to have an undesired result. Suppose that one of our very highest yielding projects is a parking lot. For a total investment of $100,000, we expect to earn a return of $40,000 a year for the next 40 years. The IRR on that project is 40%. Alternatively, we can build a medical office building on the same site. For an investment of $20,000,000 we expect to earn $6,000,000 a year for 40 years, or an IRR of 30%. We can either use the site for the parking lot or the building, but not both. Our other projects have an IRR of 20%.

If we build the parking lot because of its high IRR, and therefore bypass the building, we wind up investing $100,000 at 40% and $19,900,000 at 20% instead of $20,000,000 at 30%. This is not an optimal result. We would be better off to bypass the high-yielding parking lot and invest the entire $20,000,000 at 30%. Our decision should be based on calculating our weighted average IRR for all projects that we accept.

Excel Template

Templates 20–23 may be used to calculate present values, future values, NPVs, and internal rates of return, respectively, using your data. These templates are on the Web at www.jbpub.com.

SUMMARY

Capital budgeting represents one of the most important areas of financial management. In essence, the entire future of the organization is on the line. If projects are undertaken that don't yield adequate rates of return, they will have serious long-term consequences for the organization's profitability—and even for its viability.

To adequately evaluate projects, discounted cash flow techniques should be employed. The two most common of these methods are NPV and IRR. The essential ingredient of both of these methods is that they consider the time value of money. A nonfinancial manager doesn't necessarily have to be able to compute present values. It is vital, however, that all managers understand that *when* money is received or paid can have just as dramatic an impact on the organization as the amount received or paid.

KEY CONCEPTS

Capital budgeting—Analysis of long-term projects with respect to risk and profitability.

Net cash flow—The difference between cash receipts and cash disbursements. Cash flow is more useful than net income for project evaluation because net income fails to consider the time value of money.

Time value of money—Other things being equal, we would always prefer to receive cash sooner and pay cash later. This is because cash can be invested and earn a return in exchange for its use.

Compounding—Calculation of the return on a project, including the return earned on cash flows generated during the life of the project.

Discounting—A reversal of the compounding process. Discounting allows us to determine what a future cash flow is worth today.

Annuities—Cash flows of equal amounts, paid or received at evenly spaced periods of time, such as weekly, monthly, or annually.

Project Evaluation

Payback—A method that assesses how long it will take to receive enough cash from a project to recover the cash invested in that project.

Discounted cash flow (DCF) analysis—Methods that consider the time value of money in evaluating projects.

a. *Net present value*—Method determining whether a project earns more than a particular desired rate of return, also called the hurdle or required rate of return. The hurdle rate is based on a return for the use of money over time, plus a return for risks inherent in the project.

b. *Internal rate of return* (IRR)—Method that finds the specific rate of return on a project is expected to earn.

TEST YOUR KNOWLEDGE

See www.jbpub.com/catalog/0763726753/supplements.htm.

CHAPTER 16

Capital Structure: Long-Term Debt and Equity Financing

Organizations need resources to be able to buy land, buildings, equipment, and supplies. The money needed to acquire these assets is referred to as the organization's *capital*. Where does an organization get the capital it needs to operate? Once the organization is well established, capital can come at least partly from profits. But reinvestment of profits may not provide enough resources for everything the organization wants to do. And during the early life of any organization, other sources of capital are essential.

The dominant sources of capital are stock issuance or charitable donations, referred to as *equity financing*, or loans, referred to as *debt financing*. The choices made with respect to obtaining resources determine the *capital structure* of the organization. The capital structure of the organization, therefore, represents the right-hand side of the balance sheet: liabilities (the debt financing) and net assets or stockholder's equity (the equity financing). Clearly, charitable giving and stock issuance don't often go together. In the case of the for-profit health care organizations they have access to the stock markets, but in all likelihood very little or no access to funds via charitable gifts. On the other hand, not-for-profit health care organizations may not issue stock, but do have access to contributions and charitable giving.

CHARITABLE GIVING

For many not-for-profit health care organizations, charitable giving is a major source of capital. In fact, some health care organizations would not exist without charitable giving. It is important to note, however, that charitable giving does not come free. The old saying, "There is no such thing as a free lunch" comes to mind. Organizations must devote resources (often in the form of a staffed development office) to secure charitable gifts. Often, gifts come with donor restrictions. These restrictions may tie the hands of management in ways that do not necessarily make the most financial sense. The point of all of this is simply to note that when thinking about sources of capital, charitable gifts are an option for not-for-profit health care organizations, but require management to make carefully calculated decisions about pros and cons, just as they would do when seeking financing from the stock market or from loans, as discussed below.

COMMON STOCK

A dominant source of capital in the early life of many for-profit organizations is the issuance of *common stock*. Common stockholders own a share of the corporation's assets, have the right to vote to elect the board of directors, are entitled to a proportionate share of distributions (such as dividends), and can freely sell their ownership interest. Common stockholders invest their money, hoping to benefit from dividends and/or increases in the value of the stock.

Once a company is well established, common stock is often issued as a result of mergers (where we pay for the acquired company with stock) or to managers as a result of various compensation arrangements. However, common stock is generally not used to raise capital at that point because of the potential to dilute the share of the company owned by the current owners.

Dividends are paid to shareholders of common stock if the corporation decides to distribute some of its profits directly to its owners. Alternatively, the corporation may retain some or all of its profits for reinvestment in other potentially profitable opportunities. Hopefully this results in even greater future profits. If so, the value of each share of stock may rise, and the stockholder will be able to sell the stock for a higher price, resulting in a profit referred to as a *capital gain*.

A significant advantage the corporation gains by issuing common stock is that there are no requirements to make payments to the stockholders. If the corporation has a bad year, at least it doesn't have to worry about getting cash to make required payments to the common stockholders. A second significant advantage gained by issuing common stock is that it creates an equity base. This provides a safety cushion for lenders and makes it possible for the company to incur debt.

The issuance of common stock is not an available option for not-for-profit health care organizations. The premise of the IRS code granting tax-exempt status is the fact that these organizations are formed with the "community" as the owner with no provision for individual ownership nor any provision for the distribution of profits.

DEBT

Debt is a second major source of financing. Debt represents a loan. The borrower must pay interest and repay the amount borrowed. For an organization to be stable, a substantial portion of the organization's debt is generally in the form of long-term debt. This avoids the potential problems created if, for example, a building is financed with a 1-year loan that it intends to renew each year. What if the lender decides not to renew the loan when it comes due for payment? Long-term debt also eliminates the risk of interest rates being substantially higher when it is time to renew the loan.

Long-term debt is often issued in the form of a bond. A *bond* is a debt instrument in which investors (bondholders) lend money to the organization in exchange for the right to receive periodic (usually semi-annual) interest payments of a set amount on set dates, plus repayment of principal at a maturity date. Bondholders can sell their bonds to other investors in the same way that stock may be sold. Failure to meet these obligations puts the organization at peril of bankruptcy. For-profit health care organizations have the added benefit that interest payments on debt are tax deductible. This tax treatment lessens the effective cost of debt to the organization.

PREFERRED STOCK

For-profit health care organizations have a third potential source of capital—preferred stock. Preferred stock is a hybrid with characteristics of both stock and debt. It is part of stockholders' equity. However, in most respects it is like a bond. The dividends to preferred stockholders are paid at a predetermined rate, much like the interest rate on a bond. Unlike interest on a bond, the dividends are not tax deductible to the corporation. Why include preferred stock in a corporation's capital structure if the payments are not deductible? The dividend payments may be deferred. When a corporation falls on hard times, it still must pay the interest due on bonds. It does not have to pay the dividends due on the preferred stock. However, dividends on preferred stock must be paid before any dividends may be paid to common shareholders. Some preferred stock is cumulative and some is not. With cumulative preferred stock, any dividends that have been skipped in prior years must be paid to the preferred stockholders before dividends may be paid to common shareholders. Preferred stock is often used as part of complex financing arrangements.

COST OF CAPITAL

The choice of the relative mix of capital is an important one. For-profit health care organizations must choose between stock and debt, and not-for-profit health care organizations must choose between debt and charitable giving. In a for-profit setting, if the organization is making healthy profits, greater amounts of debt result in higher earnings per share of common stock (earnings are high and the amount of stock outstanding is low). And although this may be seen as positive, greater amounts of debt substantially increase the risk if profits start to decline. This is because interest payments must be made in good years and in bad years. If an organization doesn't have enough money to pay the interest that is due in bad years, it may be forced into bankruptcy, and may cease to exist.

Managers should try to strive for a capital structure that keeps the organization's cost of capital low. The *cost of capital* is the weighted average of the cost of common stock, preferred stock, debt, and charitable giving. The cost of debt is the interest rate that we have to pay on that debt. The cost of preferred stock is the required dividend payment. The cost of common stock is the dividend plus the growth in the value of the stock. Many organizations assume that charitable giving has no cost. But in reality, unless a donor simply walks up and hands over cash, there is always a cost associated with charitable giving. The resources used to solicit, accept, and account for charitable giving are resources that could have gone elsewhere within the organization or been invested in an interest-bearing account. Table 16-1 shows the weighted average cost of capital for Keepuwell Clinic.

The unrestricted net assets category represents a combination of unrestricted donations and also the retained earnings that the organization has that can be used for new projects. That is, as the organization earns profits over time, assets rise, and unrestricted net assets rise. Those unrestricted net assets, which represent the earnings that have been retained in the organization, become part of its capital structure. The restricted net assets represent charitable giving that is either temporarily or permanently restricted in how it may be used. The costs of these categories of capital are often estimated as the cost of what the organization could earn with an outside

Table 16-1   Weighted Average Cost of Capital

Capital	Proportion of Total Capital	Estimated Cost of Capital	Weighted Cost of Capital
Long-Term Debt	70%	8%	5.6%
Net Assets			
Unrestricted	10%	6%	0.6%
Restricted	20%	6%	1.2%
Weighted Average Cost of Capital			7.4%

investment. The weighted average cost of capital can ultimately be used by the organization to determine the hurdle rates for new project analysis (discussed in Chapter 15). By using the cost of capital as the hurdle rate, the organization isolates the financing decision from the decision to undertake a particular project relative to another project.

In for-profit health care organizations, a reasonable level of debt tends to reduce the cost of capital.

Not only does it provide the opportunity for increased profits for common shareholders, but the interest payments, as noted above, are tax deductible. This tax benefit substantially reduces the cost of debt relative to equity financing. On the other hand, one must always keep in mind the increase in financial risk caused by having debt. Further, if debt levels rise too high, lenders will be reluctant to provide further financing and the cost of debt will rise.

Table 16-2 shows two cost of capital scenarios in a for-profit version of the Keepuwell Clinic. Notice that equity capital brings with it a higher cost due to the higher risk and less favorable tax treatment relative to debt. As the level of debt increases, the cost of capital therefore goes down.

OTHER ELEMENTS OF CAPITAL STRUCTURE

In addition to common stock, preferred stock, and debt, there are several other instruments that have a place in the capital structure of for-profit health care organizations. These include stock options, stock rights, warrants, and convertibles.

Stock Options

Stock options give option holders the right, but not the obligation, to purchase shares of stock at some predetermined price over some specified period of time. Such options are often issued to key employees in an organization to motivate them to help the organization achieve or exceed its goals. For example, suppose that the corporation's common stock is currently selling for $100 a share. The owners of the stock would certainly like that value to increase. Employees may be given options to buy shares of stock at $120 per share. The options might expire in 3 years.

These options give the employees a vested interest in seeing the price of the stock go up. If the stock price fails to exceed $120, the employees will just let the options expire. However, if the stock price rises to

Table 16-2   Weighted Average Cost of Capital in a For-Profit Organization

High Equity–Low Debt

Capital	Proportion of Total Capital	Estimated Cost of Capital	Weighted Cost of Capital
Long-Term Debt	30%	8%	2.4%
Preferred Stock	40%	10%	4.0%
Common Stock	30%	14%	4.2%
Weighted Average Cost of Capital			10.6%

Low Equity–High Debt

Capital	Proportion of Total Capital	Estimated Cost of Capital	Weighted Cost of Capital
Long-Term Debt	70%	8%	5.6%
Preferred Stock	20%	10%	2.0%
Common Stock	10%	14%	1.4%
Weighted Average Cost of Capital			9.0%

$140, they can then pay just $120 to buy a share of stock that is worth $140.

Stock Rights

At times a corporation will want to raise money through an equity offering, but avoid the high costs of hiring an underwriting firm to sell the stock to the public. They can achieve this through a *rights* offering. A stock right gives the holder the right to buy a share of stock at a stated price. Usually the stated price is somewhat less than the current market price.

Stock rights are usually offered in proportion to a stockholder's current holdings. For example, suppose you owned 2,000 shares of stock in XYZ Corporation, which has 20,000 shares outstanding in total. That means you currently own 10% of the corporation. The corporation now plans to use stock rights to issue another 4,000 shares to raise additional capital. You would be entitled to 400 rights, or 10% of the total offering. If the corporation's stock is currently selling for $100 a share, and the rights allow you to buy stock at $94 a share, you would either exercise the rights, buying the 400 shares, or you could sell your rights to someone else.

Warrants and Convertibles

Warrants are similar to stock rights, but they generally have an exercise price above the level of the current market. Warrants are often given as an inducement to investors to get them to do something the organization wants. For example, a corporation may have trouble raising debt. As an inducement to lend money to the corporation, warrants may be given to the lender.

Suppose that the corporation's stock currently sells for $10 per share. Warrants may be issued to a lender allowing it to buy a certain number of shares anytime in the next 5 years for $20 a share. Lenders do not generally share in the extreme successes of the companies they lend to. They just get earned interest and repayment of the loan. However, if this corporation's stock shoots up to $100 a share, the lender could use the warrants to buy shares for $20 and join in the success it helped cause by financing the company.

Similarly, convertible debt or convertible preferred stock is debt or preferred stock that can literally be converted into shares of common stock. This convertible feature generally allows the corporation to borrow at a lower interest rate or issue preferred stock with a lower dividend rate. The lenders or purchasers of the preferred stock will take a lower interest or dividend rate because they have the potential for large profits if the common stock rises in value.

DIVIDENDS

Some for-profit companies hold themselves out as growth companies. Growth companies generally retain all or most of their profits to use for additional, hopefully highly profitable ventures. Other companies have a policy of paying dividends to their investors on a regular basis.

Some investors prefer growth companies. By holding stock without receiving dividends, they don't have to pay tax on the dividends. Later they sell the stock, hopefully at a higher

price, and pay tax at a lower capital gains rate. And in the meantime, the company has invested the entire amount of retained earnings in ventures that are potentially more lucrative than might be available to the investor. If the investor had received dividends, some of them would have been paid in tax, leaving less for reinvestment.

Other investors, however, need dividends to pay for current living expenses. Although they could sell off a little bit of stock from time to time to raise money for such expenses, they like to receive a steady, dependable flow of income. As a result, managers must decide on the dividend policy they wish to adopt. The choice affects the potential buyers of the company's stock.

At times, a corporation issues a stock dividend. For example, there might be a 10% dividend, giving the investor 1 share for every 10 shares currently owned. Or there night be a stock split such as a two-for-one split, in which case the investor gets two new shares in exchange for each old share owned. Such dividends and splits are not substantive. If you own 1,000 out of 10,000 shares, you own 10% of the company. After a two-for-one split, you own 2,000 out of 20,000 shares. You still own exactly 10% of the company.

Stock dividends and splits are generally done for psychological purposes. First, they make you feel like you have more, even if you don't. Second, they may bring the stock price down to a more reasonable trading range. For example, if a growth company keeps growing, its shares become more and more expensive. Some individuals might be tempted to buy a stock, but might decide that its price is so high, they could only afford to buy a few shares. Instead, they buy a less expensive stock so that they own more shares.

This is illogical. They should purchase the stock of the company with the greatest percentage appreciation potential. Fifty shares of a $100 stock are more valuable than 100 shares of a $50 stock, if the $100 stock has the potential to increase by a greater percentage because of the underlying profit potential of the firm. The key should not be the number of shares, but the likely percent increase in the $5,000 investment.

Nevertheless, some companies believe that if their stock is selling for $120 per share, a three-for-one split will be beneficial. It will bring the price per share down to $40 a share. That is, a value that seems substantial, but not prohibitively expensive. These companies believe that this may attract more investors, causing the stock to rise by a greater percentage than it would have without the split.

Reverse splits are also possible. If a stock is selling for a very low price, investors might be skeptical of the value of the company. A reverse split will bring the price back up to a respectable level. For example, a stock selling at $2 a share might have a one-for-ten split that would reduce the number of shares outstanding by 90%, but raise the price per share to $20. This latter price might be more likely to attract investor interest.

Some stock exchanges also have minimum dollar prices for the stock on their exchange. Without a reverse split, a stock might be delisted, substantially reducing the ability of owners of the stock to find a liquid market when they wish to sell their stock.

GETTING CAPITAL

Understanding your desired capital structure is one thing. Getting the money is another. The capital to run a business is obtained by a variety of means. These include capital campaigns, venture capital, public stock offerings, private stock placements, debt offerings, and leasing. Each of these is discussed briefly below.

Capital Campaigns

Besides on-going development activities, many not-for-profit health care organizations engage in focused fundraising activities, usually referred to as *capital campaigns.* These campaigns are typically geared around a certain theme, such as a new building or the launching of a major new service. Often capital campaigns have extended time frames (5 years is fairly typical) and publicly announced goals. To be effective, capital campaigns need a great deal of attention and the full support of senior management. Many donors require a lot of hand holding and relationship building before they are willing to part with their money. Organizations must be willing to commit significant resources (both time and money) to have a successful capital campaign.

Venture Capital

Start-up businesses must prove that they have a potentially viable business before the general public will be willing to invest in them. However, some investors, called *venture capitalists,* will put up money called *venture capital* or *risk capital* to help a new business get started. The use of venture capital in health care has increased significantly in recent years. Nashville, Tennessee (the corporate home of HCA, the nation's largest investor-owned health care corporation) has become a hot-bed of health care venture capital and start-up firms.

If you can convince these investors that they can make a lot of money by financing your start, they can get money into your firm quickly, without the lengthy and costly process of an initial public offering of stock. In return, they generally expect that an initial public offering will take place within approximately 5 years.

Businesses often begin with *seed capital* needed to do market research and product development. Seed money is often provided by the entrepreneurs starting the business themselves, or their friends and families. Businesses may raise up to $5 million this way with minimal government registration requirements. After this point, venture capitalists are called upon to provide the *working capital* needed to acquire supplies and hire workers to start producing the product, and in some cases the *acquisition capital* to acquire plant and equipment or a going business.

Venture capitalists rely heavily on the firm's business plan in determining whether to invest in the business. Therefore, the business plan may be a critical element in determining if the venture ever gets the initial capital it needs to get off the ground.

Be aware that many liken venture capitalists to the devil. The business may be something that you have conceived of and developed. It is your baby. However, not only will the venture capitalists take a substantial financial share of your business in exchange for their investment, but they will take a major share of the control of the business as well.

Public Stock Offerings

A public stock offering is one in which shares of the company are sold to a broad range of investors to secure capital for the organization. Issuing stock to the public is costly, time consuming, and complicated. At times, general economic conditions or stock market conditions will have a bigger impact on the success or failure of your offering than the underlying worth of your company will have. On the other hand, to raise significant amounts of capital without incurring an unreasonable level of debt, a public stock offering may be required.

The first time a public stock offering takes place for a company, it is referred to as an *initial public offering*. Subsequent offerings of stock to raise additional capital are referred to as *secondary issues*. Whether you are considering an initial public offering or a secondary offering, stock offerings to the public are expensive. The costs include payments to lawyers, accountants, printers, and underwriters.

Underwriters are firms that act as general contractors. They coordinate with all of the accountants, lawyers, and brokerage firms that will initially sell the stock to investors. They help to prepare all of the documents that are legally required before stock can be sold, including a prospectus and registration statement.

Once you have "gone public," your organization has an equity base that makes it easier to borrow, broader public recognition, and increased personal net worth for the original owners of the business. On the other hand, there are ongoing reporting expenses, loss of control, and potential liability of officers for failure to comply with a complicated set of rules and regulations.

Private Placements

Given some of the complexities of public offerings, sometimes businesses issue stock through a private placement. The money received from venture capitalists is one type of private placement. Even when the amounts of capital to be raised are substantially higher—perhaps hundreds of millions of dollars or even several billion dollars—a private placement is sometime possible. Selling stock directly to a few large investors avoids much of the cost of a public offering and avoids the need to file certain elaborate documents with the government. Large insurance companies often participate in such placements, putting perhaps $50 or $100 million into a company in exchange for stock.

Private placements can also raise funds much more quickly than a public offering can. However, in most cases the amount of money that can be raised from a private placement may be substantially less than the business might raise from a public offering. It should also be noted that, because of the risks involved to the investor, government regulations tend to prohibit all but sophisticated investors from participating in such placements.

Bond Offerings

Bonds can be issued through private placements or public offerings in the same way as stocks are. As with stocks, private placements are simpler and less expensive, but don't have the ability to raise as much money as a public offering.

Bonds are a particularly good alternative to bank financing because they can be for large amounts of money, they can extend for long periods of time (typically 30 years), providing stability, and they eliminate the intermediary. For example, a bank might pay 4% to a depositor and then lend the depositor's money to a corporation for 9%. The 5% difference represents the bank's costs and profits. If the corporation issues a bond at an interest rate of 6.5%, it will pay 2.5% less than the bank charges, and the ultimate investors will receive 2.5% more than they would have received from the bank. The investors have more risk than they would if they deposited their money in the bank. The corporation has greater costs and legal compliance issues than it would if it borrowed the money from a bank. For a large loan, it is worth paying these higher costs to get a lower interest rate.

Leasing

Another source of financing is leasing. Someone buys an asset, such as a building, and rents it to a business that wants to use that asset. The business using the asset is a lessee, and the owner of the asset is a lessor. Leasing is very similar to having borrowed money and purchased the asset directly. Therefore, leases are generally considered to be a form of debt financing.

KEY CONCEPTS

Capital—The money needed by the firm to acquire resources.

Capital structure—Mix of debt and equity used to finance the firm.

>*Equity financing*—Capital provided in exchange for an ownership interest, typically through the issuance of stock.

>*Debt financing*—Capital provided in the form of loans.

Stock option—Security that gives the holder the right to purchase shares of stock at some predetermined price, usually above market value.

Stock right—Security that gives the holder the right to buy a share of stock at a stated price, usually below market value.

Sources of capital—Charitable giving, venture capital, public stock offerings, private stock placements, debt offerings, and leasing.

TEST YOUR KNOWLEDGE

See www.jbpub.com/catalog/0763726753/ supplements.htm.

CHAPTER 17

Case Study:
Happy Hospital

In this chapter we trace through the events and financial decisions of a fictitious hospital—Happy Hospital. This case study is designed to review much of the material presented in previous chapters. Obviously, no case study can cover every type of accounting event or issue. This case study does, however, provide a good overview of many of the issues faced by health care financial managers.

RECOVERING FROM NEW YEAR'S EVE: IS IT REALLY THE START OF ANOTHER YEAR?

Wow, what a night. Now that the celebrations are over, it is time to start another year at Happy Hospital. Today is January 1, 2008. Happy is a medium sized community hospital with 115 beds. We are part of a loose affiliation of six hospitals and two long-term care facilities. Happy is recognized by the IRS as a 501(c)3 Corporation and is therefore exempt from paying income taxes. Happy has a long and proud tradition of providing high-quality care, meeting the needs of the community, and serving all individuals with respect and dignity regardless of ability to pay. Tables 17-1 through 17-3 present the end of year financial statements for 2007 and

2006. (Magically, they have been prepared, audited, and certified overnight.)

WHAT SHOULD WE DO WITH ALL THAT MONEY?

In looking over the financial statements you first notice that Happy Hospital is sitting on a sizeable amount of current assets. In fact, Happy Hospital is going into the current year with approximately $12.5 million in current assets compared to $4.3 million in current liabilities. (A current ratio of 2.9!) The vast majority of the $12.5 million is in accounts receivable, but we do have just over $800,000 in cash.

The CEO of Happy Hospital, Mr. Harm O. Knee, has long been talking about the need to automate some of the medical records and move toward an electronic medical record. Given the 2007 operating loss of $829,000 (Table 17-2), he is pushing harder than ever. Perhaps it's time to invest in new technologies that can improve efficiency and help reduce medical errors. Recently two different vendors have been by to present their medical records systems. Both systems are highly regarded for automating much of the medical records process and thereby improving efficiency and reducing

Table 17-1

Happy Hospital
Statement of Financial Position
As of December 31, 2007 and December 31, 2006

	December 31	
	2007	2006
Assets		
Current Assets		
Cash and Cash Equivalents	$ 804,331	$ 105,331
Accounts Receivable		
Patients, Less Allowances for Uncollectible Accounts	8,957,621	9,608,145
Other	980,311	803,025
Total Accounts Receivable	9,937,932	10,411,170
Inventory	1,234,344	498,100
Prepaid Expenses and Other Assets	504,329	971,917
Total Current Assets	12,480,936	11,986,518
Assets Limited as to Use	55,732,204	52,233,340
Investments	1,639,529	1,464,780
Property and Equipment, Net	16,347,859	16,886,005
Prepaid Pension Asset	296,797	1,298,170
Total Assets	$ 86,497,325	$ 83,868,813
Liabilities and Net Assets		
Current Liabilities		
Accounts Payable and Accrued Expenses	$ 1,601,308	$ 1,586,144
Accrued Compensation and Amounts Withheld	2,399,365	2,491,736
Current Portion of Estimated Third-Party Payor Settlements	322,161	1,400,000
Total Current Liabilities	4,322,834	5,477,880
Estimated Third-Party Payor Settlements, Less Current Portion	3,697,939	3,530,000
Total Liabilities	8,020,773	9,007,880
Net Assets		
Unrestricted	77,478,008	73,967,293
Temporarily Restricted	798,544	693,640
Permanently Restricted	200,000	200,000
Total Net Assets	78,476,552	74,860,933
Total Liabilities and Net Assets	$ 86,497,325	$ 83,868,813

Table 17-2

Happy Hospital
Statement of Operations
As of December 31, 2007 and December 31, 2006

	Year Ended December 31	
	2007	2006
Unrestricted Revenues		
Net Patient Service Revenue	$ 51,119,826	$ 48,659,436
Other Operating Revenue	2,989,626	3,136,716
Total Unrestricted Revenues	54,109,452	51,796,152
Expenses		
Wages	49,606,566	47,076,683
Insurance	1,005,783	1,024,889
Inventory	1,275,524	1,053,367
Depreciation	442,891	421,597
Provision for Uncollectible Accounts	2,607,828	2,237,701
Total Expenses	54,938,592	51,814,237
(Loss) From Operations Before Adjustments to Prior Year Third-Party Payer Settlements and Pension Expense in Excess of Plan Contribution	(829,140)	(18,085)
Pension Expense in Excess of Plan Contribution	(1,001,373)	(451,432)
Adjustments to Prior Year Third-Party Payer Settlements	329,626	1,360,937
Operating (Loss) Income	(1,500,887)	891,420
Nonoperating Gains		
Investment Income	3,815,629	96,280
Unrestricted Gifts and Bequests	33,654	334,067
Other Miscellaneous Income	195,363	12,300
Nonoperating Gains	4,044,646	442,647
Excess of Revenues and Gains Over Expenses	2,543,759	1,334,067
Other Changes in Unrestricted Net Assets		
Changes in Net Unrealized Gain on Investments	966,956	6,431,704
Increase in Unrestricted Net Assets	$ 3,510,715	$ 7,765,771

Table 17-3

Happy Hospital
Statement of Cash Flows
As of December 31, 2007 and December 31, 2006

	Year Ended December 31	
	2007	**2006**
Operating Activities		
Increase in Net Assets	**$ 3,510,715**	$ 7,765,771
Adjustments to Reconcile Increase in Net Assets to Net Cash Provided by Operating Activities		
Depreciation	**2,561,982**	2,421,597
Net Realized and Unrealized Gains on Investments	**(3,208,808)**	(5,086,230)
Restricted Investment Income	**(34,000)**	(42,839)
Provision for Uncollectible Accounts	**2,770,044**	2,237,701
Loss on Disposal of Property and Equipment	**(23,185)**	(24,888)
Changes in Operating Assets and Liabilities		
Patient Accounts Receivable	**(2,119,520)**	(4,845,803)
Other Receivables	**(177,286)**	(360,806)
Inventory	**(736,244)**	(14,589)
Prepaid Expenses and Other Assets	**467,588**	(225,660)
Prepaid Pension Asset	**1,001,373**	451,432
Accounts Payable and Accrued Expenses	**15,164**	(284,615)
Accrued Compensation and Amounts Withheld	**(92,371)**	779,623
Estimated Third-Party Payer Settlements	**(909,900)**	—
Net Cash Provided by Operating Activities	**3,025,552**	2,770,694
Investing Activities		
Expenditures for Property and Equipment	**(2,028,551)**	(2,360,317)
Proceeds from Sales of Property and Equipment	**27,900**	55,728
Purchases of Investments, Net	**(464,805)**	(1,090,947)
Net Cash Used in Investing Activities	**(2,465,456)**	(3,395,536)
Financing Activity		
Restricted Investment Income	**34,000**	42,839
Net Cash Provided by Financing Activity	**34,000**	42,839
Increase (Decrease) in Cash and Cash Equivalents	**699,000**	(453,257)
Cash and Cash Equivalents at Beginning of Year	**105,331**	558,588
Cash and Cash Equivalents at End of Year	**$ 804,331**	$ 105,331

errors. The two systems have very different cash flow and investment requirements. Table 17-4 presents the expected cash flow for each of the two options.

As you can see, Option 1 has a lower up-front purchase price, but a higher annual maintenance cost and doesn't seem to yield as much savings down the road. From a financial standpoint, which of these options is better? It is impossible to tell at this point. Given what we learned about the time value of money, we must first find the present value of the cash flows of the two options in order to appropriately analyze them. Table 17-5 presents the net present value calculations for the two options assuming a discount rate of 10%.

It's clear from the net present value calculations that Option 2 is a better choice despite its higher up-front purchase price. The net present value for Option 2 is almost $25,000 higher than Option 1. Although Option 2 may be the "better" choice, we have to be careful. A close inspection of the components of the net present value calculations reveals that Option 2 covers its large up-front cost with projected savings from reduced errors that is almost twice as much as Option 1. The concern here might be that sometimes projected savings never materialize. The net present value calculation is only as good as the data that we put into the calculation. However, the vendor assures us that we will in fact realize those savings, so let's go ahead

Table 17-4   Expected Cash Flow for Two Medical Records Systems

Option 1

	Up-Front	Year 1	Year 2	Year 3	Year 4	Year 5
Purchase Price	$ (475,000)					
Maintenance Cost		$ (10,000)	$ (10,300)	$ (10,609)	$ (10,927)	$ (11,255)
Personnel Savings		47,500	49,400	51,376	53,431	55,568
Savings Due to Reduced Errors		75,000	86,250	99,188	114,066	131,175
Total	$ (475,000)	$ 112,500	$ 125,350	$ 139,955	$ 156,569	$ 175,489

Option 2

	Up-Front	Year 1	Year 2	Year 3	Year 4	Year 5
Purchase Price	$ (700,000)					
Maintenance Cost		$ (5,000)	$ (5,150)	$ (5,305)	$ (5,464)	$ (5,628)
Personnel Savings		24,500	25,480	26,499	27,559	28,662
Savings Due to Reduced Errors		140,000	161,000	185,150	212,923	244,861
Total	$ (700,000)	$ 159,500	$ 181,330	$ 206,345	$ 235,018	$ 267,895

Table 17-5   Net Present Value Calculations for Two Medical Records Systems

Option 1

	Up-Front	Year 1	Year 2	Year 3	Year 4	Year 5
Purchase Price	$(475,000)					
Maintenance Cost		$ (10,000)	$ (10,300)	$ (10,609)	$ (10,927)	$ (11,255)
Personnel Savings		47,500	49,400	51,376	53,431	55,568
Savings Due to Reduced Errors		75,000	86,250	99,188	114,066	131,175
Total	$(475,000)	$ 112,500	$ 125,350	$ 139,955	$ 156,569	$ 175,489
	$ 102,273 ◄					
	103,595 ◄					
	105,150 ◄					
	106,939 ◄					
	108,965 ◄					
Total Present Value Years 1–5	$ 526,921					
Net Present Value	**$ 51,921**					

Option 2

	Up-Front	Year 1	Year 2	Year 3	Year 4	Year 5
Purchase Price	$(700,000)					
Maintenance Cost		$ (5,000)	$ (5,150)	$ (5,305)	$ (5,464)	$ (5,628)
Personnel Savings		24,500	25,480	26,499	27,559	28,662
Savings Due to Reduced Errors		140,000	161,000	185,150	212,923	244,861
Total	$(700,000)	$ 159,500	$ 181,330	$ 206,345	$ 235,018	$ 267,895
	$ 145,000 ◄					
	149,860 ◄					
	155,030 ◄					
	160,520 ◄					
	166,342 ◄					
Total Present Value Years 1–5	$ 776,751					
Net Present Value	**$ 76,751**					

and commit to the Option 2 system. The purchase of this system will in fact be our first financial transaction for this fiscal year. Assume that sufficient money was budgeted for this purchase when our budgets for this year were approved late last year. Let's take a look at what else we are going to do this year.

WHAT A BUSY YEAR! TRACKING FINANCIAL EVENTS

Not all of our decisions and transactions involve large sums of money like our new electronic medical record system. In fact, the vast majority of financial events are relatively small routine events that must be tracked throughout the year. Below is a list of all the transactions recorded on our books during the year. As you can see, our new electronic medical record system from above is the very first transaction.

1. Happy Hospital purchased a new electronic medical record system. This purchase was made with $700,000 in cash.
2. Happy Hospital took out a long-term loan in the amount of $1,500,000.
3. Happy Hospital purchased inventory on account costing $766,700.
4. Happy Hospital billed patients a total of $20,756,800 (net of contractual allowances and charity care). Of this amount, they assume that 3% will be bad debt.
5. Happy Hospital purchased a new piece of equipment for $84,000 cash.
6. Happy Hospital paid $347,210 of their accounts payable.
7. Happy Hospital's workers earned $27,567,126 in wages. Happy paid $25,167,761 and owed the balance.
8. Inventory previously purchased for $954,000 was used.

9. Happy Hospital purchased a 1-year malpractice policy for $1,398,755 in cash.
10. Happy Hospital received a gift in the form of property from their independently wealthy founder Mrs. R.U. Happy. The property is valued at $550,000 and has no restrictions.
11. Six months into the year, Happy Hospital contracted with a managed care organization to provide services to a pool of 90,000 covered lives for 1 year. The managed care company has paid in advance the full annual premium of $3,900,000.
12. Happy Hospital charged and billed the non-managed care patients another $32,378,900. Of this amount, they assume that 3% will be bad debt.
13. Happy Hospital paid $614,532 of their accounts payable.
14. Happy Hospital accrued wages payable in the amount of $24,567,555. Of this amount Happy Hospital paid $19,542,765.
15. Cash collections from patient accounts were $46,756,321.
16. Happy Hospital made a payment on their long-term loan in the amount of $72,200. This included $62,700 of interest and $9,500 of principal.

Table 17-6 shows how each of the listed transactions impacts the balance sheet equation. (Table 17-6 is also available as an Excel file at www.jbpub.com.) The first line of figures within the table is the beginning balance for each account (see Table 17-1). Each subsequent line demonstrates how each specific transaction impacts the balance sheet equation. For example, in transaction 6, Happy Hospital paid its suppliers $347,210. Cash goes down by this amount and in addition, accounts payable goes down. Remember, assets must always equal liabilities plus net assets.

Table 17-6   Tracking the Financial Transactions

	Cash	Accounts Receivable	Other	Inventory	Prepaid Expenses	Assets— Limited Use	Invest- ments	Property, Plant and Equipment, Net	Prepaid Pension Asset
Beginning Balance	$ 804,331	$ 8,957,621	$980,311	$1,234,344	$ 504,329	$55,732,204	$1,639,529	$16,347,859	$296,797
1 New Equipment	(700,000)							700,000	
2 New Long-Term Debt	1,500,000								
3 Inventory on Account				766,700					
4 Patient Services		20,756,800							
Provision for Bad Debt		(622,704)							
5 New Equipment	(84,000)							84,000	
6 Payments	(347,210)								
7 Paid Wages	(25,167,761)								
8 Inventory Expense				(954,000)					
9 Malpractice Insurance	(1,398,755)				1,398,755				
10 Gift								550,000	
11 Managed Care Contract	3,900,000								
12 Patient Services		32,378,900							
Provision for Bad Debt		(971,367)							
13 Payments	(614,532)								
14 Accrued Wages									
Paid Wages	(19,542,765)								
15 Collections	46,756,321	(46,756,321)							
16 Loan Payment—Interest	(62,700)								
Loan Payment—Principal	(9,500)								
Ending Balance	$ 5,033,429	$13,742,929	$980,311	$1,047,044	$1,903,084	$55,732,204	$1,639,529	$17,681,859	$296,797

TIME TO CLOSE THE BOOKS

Now that all the transactions have been recorded is it time to take the balance of each account and create the financial statements? No. There are still a number of financial adjustments that must be made to the books before we can create the financial statements. Happy Hospital has a number of common adjustments to be made at this time. First, Happy Hospital must take the annual depreciation expense associated with its property, plant, and equipment (PPE). Let's assume that the PPE that was on the books prior to this year has a current depreciation of $457,654. In addition, however, we must remember that we purchased

two pieces of equipment this year. The electronic medical record system for $700,000 has a useful life of 10 years and no salvage value. The hospital plans on using the straight-line method for calculating depreciation. Therefore, this year's depreciation amount for this equipment is $70,000.

The second piece of equipment was $84,000. It has a useful life of 4 years and a salvage value of $2,500. This asset, however, will be used up in a very different rate and therefore, Happy Hospital will use the Double Declining Balance Method for calculating depreciation. Based on this approach, the current depreciation is $42,000 (Depreciable Base $\times 2/n = \$84,000 \times 2/4 = \$42,000$, where n is the number of years we expect to

Table 17-6 Tracking the Financial Transactions *(continued)*

=	Accounts Payable	Accrued Compensation	Unearned Revenue	Current Portion of 3rd-party Payer Settlements	Estimated 3rd-party Payer Settlements —Noncurrent	Long-Term + Debt	Unrestricted Net Assets	Temporarily Restricted Net Assets	Permanently Restricted Net Assets
	$ 1,601,308	$ 2,399,365	$ 0	$322,161	$3,697,939	$ 0	$77,478,008	$798,544	$200,000
						1,500,000			
	766,700								
							20,756,800		
							(622,704)		
	(347,210)								
		2,399,365					(27,567,126)		
							(954,000)		
							550,000		
			3,900,000						
							32,378,900		
							(971,367)		
	(614,532)								
		24,567,555					(24,567,555)		
		(19,542,765)							
							(62,700)		
						(9,500)			
	$1,406,$266	$ 9,823,520	$3,900,000	$322,161	$3,697,939	$1,490,500	$76,418,256	$798,544	$200,000

use the equipment). The three depreciations (for PPE owned prior to this year and the two acquisitions made this year) must be combined to come up with the annual depreciation expense. In this case, the depreciation expense is $569,654. This transaction is listed as number 17 in Table 17-7.

Remember that managed care contract that Happy Hospital received in the middle of the year? The next adjustment is to recognize the fact that 6 months have gone by since we received the annual payment from the managed care company. In this case, we received the cash, but had yet to deliver any service, so we created a $3,900,000 unearned revenue liability. To recognize that 6 months of the contract has expired, we must

reduce the liability (we no longer are obligated to provide 6 months worth of care) and recognize the revenue. This adjustment is listed as number 18 in Table 17-7.

Once we have recognized any unearned revenue we must turn our attention to adjusting any prepaid expenses that we made during the year. If you recall, we purchased 1 year's worth of malpractice insurance during the year. This insurance reduced cash (we paid for the full year up-front) and added to the prepaid expenses balance. (The insurance policy is an asset until we use it up, at which point it will become an expense.) Let's assume that we purchased the policy on March 1. The adjustment is therefore to recognize that we have used up 10 months of

Table 17-7   Final Adjustments

	Cash	Accounts Receivable	Other	Inventory	Prepaid Expenses	Assets— Limited Use	Invest- ments	Property, Plant and Equipment, Net	Prepaid Pension Asset
Beginning Balance	$ 804,331	$ 8,957,621	$980,311	$1,234,344	$ 504,329	$55,732,204	$1,639,529	$16,347,859	$296,797
1 New Equipment	(700,000)							700,000	
2 New Long-Term Debt	1,500,000								
3 Inventory on Account				766,700					
4 Patient Services		20,756,800							
Provision for Bad Debt		(622,704)							
5 New Equipment	(84,000)							84,000	
6 Payments	(347,210)								
7 Paid Wages	(25,167,761)								
8 Inventory Expense				(954,000)					
9 Malpractice Insurance	(1,398,755)				1,398,755				
10 Gift								550,000	
11 Managed Care Contract	3,900,000								
12 Patient Services		32,378,900							
Provision for Bad Debt		(971,367)							
13 Payments	(614,532)								
14 Accrued Wages									
Paid Wages	(19,542,765)								
15 Collections	46,756,321	(46,756,321)							
16 Loan Payment—Interest	(62,700)								
Loan Payment—Principal	(9,500)								
17 Depreciation								(569,654)	
18 Revenue Recognition									
19 Expense Recognition					(1,165,629)				
Ending Balance	$ 5,033,429	$13,742,929	$980,311	$1,047,044	$ 737,455	$55,732,204	$1,639,529	$17,112,205	$296,797

the 12-month policy. The annual cost was $1,398,755 so 10/12 of this is $1,165,629. The adjustment to recognize the expense is shown in Table 17-7 as transaction 19.

PUTTING TOGETHER THE END-OF-YEAR FINANCIAL STATEMENTS

Now that all the transactions have been recorded and the year-end adjustments have been made, it is time to put together the end-of-year financial statements. Given the balance sheet equation we have maintained over the course of the year, creating the statement of financial position (the balance sheet) will be relatively straightforward.

The bottom line of Table 17-7 is in fact the end-of-year statement of financial position. Table 17-8 presents the formal statement for Happy Hospital at the end of 2008. Using the changes to net assets during the year from Table 17-7, Table 17-9 presents the Statement of Operations. In Table 17-10, we present the Statement of Cash Flows using the indirect method.

HOW DID WE DO? USING RATIO ANALYSIS

Well, it is almost time for another New Year's Eve party. But before we leave for the holiday, we should probably look at how we did dur-

Table 17-7 Final Adjustments *(continued)*

=	Accounts Payable	Accrued Compensation	Unearned Revenue	Current Portion of 3rd-party Payer Settlements	Estimated 3rd-party Payer Settlements —Noncurrent	Long-Term Debt	+	Unrestricted Net Assets	Temporarily Restricted Net Assets	Permanently Restricted Net Assets
	$ 1,601,308	$ 2,399,365	$ 0	$322,161	$3,697,939	$ 0		$77,478,008	$798,544	$200,000
						1,500,000				
	766,700									
								20,756,800		
								(622,704)		
	(347,210)									
		2,399,365						(27,567,126)		
								(954,000)		
								550,000		
			3,900,000							
								32,378,900		
								(971,367)		
	(614,532)									
		24,567,555						(24,567,555)		
		(19,542,765)								
								(62,700)		
						(9,500)				
								(569,654)		
			(1,950,000)					1,950,000		
								(1,165,629)		
	$1,406,$266	$ 9,823,520	$1,950,000	$322,161	$3,697,939	$1,490,500		$76,632,973	$798,544	$200,000

ing the past year. Using our financial statements, we can now prepare a complete set of financial ratios and assess our performance and our current position. Table 17-11 shows the major ratios presented in Chapter 13.

As you can see, our days cash on hand has increased from 5.66 days in 2007 to 33.82 days in 2008. However, that doesn't mean that we can assume our liquidity position is better. Note that our current ratio fell from 2.89 to 1.60 and our quick ratio fell from 2.49 to 1.46. Here we have clearly conflicting evidence about our liquidity. This points out the need to review a lot of information about an organization before drawing a conclusion about its financial position.

The efficiency ratios raise a number of cautions. The days in accounts payable is only 9.18 for 2008, but that doesn't tell the whole story. Look at the difference between our average payment period and our days in accounts payables. This difference must be due to the large accrued compensation figures that are included in the average payment period ratio, but not in the days in accounts payable figure. Happy Hospital is keeping current on their payment to suppliers, but appears to be keeping employees waiting. This could be a sign of trouble. The other interesting figure is the days in accounts receivables. Over the past year, we have taken an additional 30 days to collect

Table 17-8

Happy Hospital
Statement of Financial Position
As of December 31, 2008 and December 31, 2007

	December 31	
	2008	2007
Assets		
Current Assets		
Cash and Cash Equivalents	$ 5,033,429	$ 804,331
Accounts Receivable		
Patients, Less Allowances for Uncollectible Accounts	13,742,929	8,957,621
Other	980,311	980,311
Total Accounts Receivable	14,723,240	9,937,932
Inventory	1,047,044	1,234,344
Prepaid Expenses and Other Assets	737,455	504,329
Total Current Assets	21,541,168	12,480,936
Assets Limited as to Use	55,732,204	55,732,204
Investments	1,639,529	1,639,529
Property and Equipment, Net	17,112,205	16,347,859
Prepaid Pension Asset	296,797	296,797
Total Assets	$ 96,321,903	$ 86,497,325
Liabilities and Net Assets		
Current Liabilities		
Accounts Payable and Accrued Expenses	$ 1,406,266	$ 1,601,308
Accrued Compensation and Amounts Withheld	9,823,520	2,399,365
Unearned Revenue	1,950,000	0
Current Portion of Estimated Third-Party Payer Settlements	322,161	322,161
Total Current Liabilities	13,501,947	4,322,834
Estimated Third-Party Payor Settlements, Less Current Portion	3,697,93	3,697,939
Long-Term Debt	1,490,500	0
Total Liabilities	5,188,439	8,020,773
Net Assets		
Unrestricted	76,632,973	77,478,008
Temporarily Restricted	798,544	798,544
Permanently Restricted	200,000	200,000
Total Net Assets	77,631,517	78,476,552
Total Liabilities and Net Assets	$ 96,321,903	$ 86,497,325

Table 17-9

Happy Hospital
Statement of Operations
As of December 31, 2008 and December 31, 2007

	Year Ended December 31	
	2008	**2007**
Unrestricted Revenues		
Net Patient Service Revenue	$ 53,135,700	$ 51,119,826
Other Operating Revenue	1,950,000	2,989,626
Total Unrestricted Revenues	55,085,700	54,109,452
Expenses		
Wages	52,134,681	49,606,566
Insurance	1,165,629	1,005,783
Inventory	954,000	1,275,524
Interest	62,700	0
Depreciation	569,654	442,891
Provision for Uncollectible Accounts	1,594,071	2,607,828
Total Expenses	56,480,735	54,938,592
Gain/(Loss) from Operations Before Adjustments to Prior Year Third-Party Payer Settlements and Pension Expense in Excess of Plan Contribution	(1,395,035)	(829,140)
Pension Expense in Excess of Plan Contribution	0	(1,001,373)
Adjustments to Prior Year Third-Party Payer Settlements	0	329,626
Operating (Loss) Income	(1,395,035)	(1,500,887)
Nonoperating Gains		
Investment Income	0	3,815,629
Unrestricted Gifts and Bequests	550,000	33,654
Other Miscellaneous Income	0	195,363
Nonoperating Gains	550,000	4,044,646
Excess of Revenues and Gains Over Expenses	(845,035)	2,543,759
Other Changes in Unrestricted Net Assets		
Changes in Net Unrealized Gain on Investments	0	966,956
Increase in Unrestricted Net Assets	$ (845,035)	$ 3,510,715

Table 17-10

Happy Hospital
Statement of Cash Flows
As of December 31, 2008 and December 31, 2007

	Year Ended December 31	
	2008	**2007**
Operating Activities		
Increase/(Decrease) in Net Assets	$ (845,035)	$ 3,510,715
Adjustments to Reconcile Increase (Decrease) in Net Assets to Net Cash Provided by Operating Activities		
Depreciation	569,654	2,561,982
Net Realized and Unrealized Gains on Investments	—	(3,208,808)
Restricted Investment Income	—	(34,000)
Provision for Uncollectible Accounts	1,594,071	2,770,044
Loss on Disposal of Property and Equipment	—	(23,185)
Gain on Capital Gift	(550,000)	—
Changes in Operating Assets and Liabilities		
Patient Accounts Receivable	(6,379,379)	(2,119,520)
Other Receivables	—	(177,286)
Inventory	187,300	(736,244)
Prepaid Expenses and Other Assets	(233,126)	467,588
Prepaid Pension Asset	—	1,001,373
Accounts Payable and Accrued Expenses	(195,042)	15,164
Accrued Compensation and Amounts Withheld	7,424,155	(92,371)
Unearned Revenue	1,950,000	—
Estimated Third-Party Payer Settlements	—	(909,900)
Net Cash Provided by Operating Activities	3,522,598	3,025,552
Investing Activities		
Expenditures for Property and Equipment	(784,000)	(2,028,551)
Proceeds from Sales of Property and Equipment	—	27,900
Purchases of Investments, Net	—	(464,805)
Net Cash Used in Investing Activities	(784,000)	(2,465,456)
Financing Activity		
Loan Proceeds	1,500,000	—
Loan Repayment	(9,500)	—
Restricted Investment Income	—	34,000
Net Cash Provided by Financing Activity	1,490,500	34,000
Increase (Decrease) in Cash and Cash Equivalents	4,229,098	699,000
Cash and Cash Equivalents at Beginning of Year	804,331	105,331
Cash and Cash Equivalents at End of Year	$ 5,033,429	$ 804,331

Table 7-11

Happy Hospital
Financial Ratios
For the Years 2008 and 2007

	2008	2007
Liquidity		
Current Ratio	1.60	2.89
Quick ratio	1.46	2.49
Days Cash on Hand	33.82	5.66
Efficiency		
Days in Accounts Receivables	97.56	67.04
Days in Accounts Payable	9.18	10.73
Average Payment Period	88.14	28.95
Total Asset Turnover	0.57	0.63
Solvency		
Interest Coverage	−12.48	NA
Debt Service Coverage	−2.95	NA
Long-Term Debt to Net Assets	0.02	0.00
Profitability		
Total Margin	−0.02	0.06
Operating Margin	−0.03	−0.02
Return on Assets	−0.01	−0.01
Return on Net Assets	−0.02	−0.01

payment from our customers! This is certainly worthy of our attention (after the New Year's Eve party).

The solvency and profitability numbers all reflect the fact that we have had 2 difficult income years. As you may have noticed, Happy Hospital did not have any debt coming into 2008. They did take on some long-term debt this year. Because the hospital lost money, they have negative interest and debt service coverage ratios. Also, all of the profitability ratios are negative as Happy Hospital had both operating and total losses for the year. Clearly there are serious signs of financial stress, and we have our work cut out for us to turn around the 2 years of operating losses.

Index

B